TESTS
Chinese Acupuncture and Moxibustion

Dr. Cui Yongqiang, M.D., and Dr. Chen Ken, M.D.

FOREIGN LANGUAGES PRESS

First Edition 1993
Third Printing 2001

I dedicate this book to my daughter, Yi Xin, whose name in Chinese means "the flourishing of Yi Yi" (the herbal plant Coix).

Cui Yongqiang

Dec. 15. 1999

English text edited by Kenneth Lubowich

Special thanks to Ms. Della Estrada of the United States: for her help in re-editing this book.

Home Page:
http: //www.flp.com.cn
E-mail Addresses:
info@flp.com.cn
Sales@flp.com.cn

ISBN 7-119-01587-7

Published by Foreign Languages Press
24 Baiwanzhuang Road, Beijing 100037, China
Distributed by China International Book Trading Corporation
35 Chegongzhuang Xilu, Beijing 100044, China
P.O. Box 399, Beijing, China
Printed in the People's Republic of China

Preface

The TCM (traditional Chinese medicine) education and examination programme is sponsored by the China Academy of Traditional Chinese Medicine.

Entrusted by the World Health Organization (WHO), the Ministry of Public Health of the People's Republic of China sponsored its first formal acupuncture training course for foreign doctors in 1981 and from then on, normalized TCM education and examinations began to spread worldwide.

This selection of examination questions in TCM is offered in the hope that it may be found useful in any of the following four ways:

1. As a source of ready-made questions for use by examiners of TCM-related organizations.

2. As a source of ideas which may aid examiners in the construction of new questions.

3. As an aid to candidates planning to take TCM examinations and to score high on them.

4. As a means by which students can assess their own progress in acquiring TCM knowledge.

The questions in this book will show you what is required and therefore help you get the most out of your studies. You will also get the "feel" of the examination. This book contains many "similar situations" —as you will discover when you take the actual examinations in China and abroad.

In going over the questions in this book, you will not—if you use this book properly—be satisfied merely with the answer to a particular question. You will want to do additional study on the other choices for the same questions. In this way you will broaden your background, which will help your preparation for the examination or your treatment of the patients.

Included in this book are multiple-choice and traditional questions, both focusing on the mastery of basic TCM theory, acupuncture and manipulations, diagnosis and case analysis. There is now growing evidence to suggest that these questions appear simultaneously in all kinds of examinations, as are being demonstrated daily in China.

The answers appear at the back and, where available, a figure is provided showing the facility of the question. This is derived from the average proportion of candidates correctly answering the question over all the occasions when it has been used in formal examinations. It has to be emphasized also that all the answers involved in this book do not go far from the textbooks *Essentials of Chinese Acupuncture* and *Chinese Acupuncture and Moxibustion* published by Foreign Languages Press.

If you would like further information on TCM training courses[1] please write me at: Guanganmen Hospital, China Academy of Traditional Chinese Medicine, Beijing 100053, China[2].

Dr. Cui Yongqiang, M.D.
International Clinical TCM Training Centre,
Guanganmen Hospital,
China Academy of Traditional Chinese Medicine
Collaborating Centre of Traditional Medicine
World Health Organization (WHO)

Dec, 15, 1999

1. A newly opened TCM consulting system(specially designed for advanced practitioners of TCM) through the internet.
2. You may also email me at: cuiyongq@public. fhnet. cn.net

CONTENTS

Part One Multiple-choice Questions

"A" Type Questions 1
I. Yin-Yang and the Five Elements 1
II. Zang-Fu, Qi, Blood and Body Fluid 7
III. The Channels, Collaterals and Acupoints 15
IV. Diagnostic Methods 37
V. Differentiation of Syndromes 46
VI. Techniques of Acupuncture, Moxibustion and Cupping 59
VII. Treatment of Diseases 64
Solutions to the Exercises 98

"B" Type Questions 99
I. Yin-Yang and the Five Elements 100
II. Zang-Fu, Qi, Blood and Body Fluid 101
III. The Channels, Collaterals and Acupoints 103
IV. Diagnostic Methods 105
V. Differentiation of Syndromes 109
VI. Techniques of Acupuncture, Moxibustion and Cupping 114
VII. Treatment of Diseases 115
Solutions to the Exercises 120

"C" Type Questions 120
I. Yin-Yang and the Five Elements 121
II. Zang-Fu, Qi, Blood and Body Fluid 122
III. The Channels, Collaterals and Acupoints 123
IV. Diagnostic Methods 123
V. Differentiation of Syndromes 124
VI. Techniques of Acupuncture, Moxibustion and Cupping 126

VII. Treatment of Diseases 127
Solutions to the Exercises 129

"K" Type Questions 130
I. Yin-Yang and the Five Elements 130
II. Zang-Fu, Qi, Blood and Body Fluid 134
III. The Channels, Collaterals and Acupoints 140
IV. Diagnostic Methods 149
V. Differentiation of Syndromes 160
VI. Techniques of Acupuncture, Moxibustion and Cupping 170
VII. Treatment of Diseases 173
Solutions to the Exercises 181

Part Two Traditional Questions

I. Underline the Part of the Statement Which Is Incorrect 183
Solutions to the Exercises 184
II. True or False 184
Solutions to the Exercises 187
III. Fill the Blanks 187
Solutions to the Exercises 193
IV. Definitions of TCM Terms 194
V. Case Analysis 197
VI. Questions and Answers 207

Appendixes

Standard Acupuncture Nomenclature (Part 1 Revised Edition) 224
Standard Acupuncture Nomenclature (Part 2 Revised Edition) 231

About the Authors

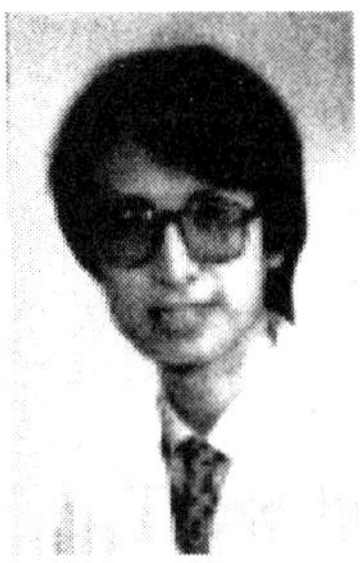

Dr. Cui Yongqiang, a graduate from the Beijing University of Traditional Chinese Medicine, is now teaching at the International Clinical Acupuncture Training Centre (a cooperative TCM centre entrusted by the World Health Organization), Guanganmen Hospital, China Academy of Traditional Chinese Medicine. He is the first Chinese doctor to devote himself to the standardization of tests of Chinese acupuncture and moxibustion. Years of experience in supervising foreign students have enabled him to write this book. He is also the co-author of Handbook to Chinese Auricular Therapy, published by Foreign Languages Press in 1991[1].

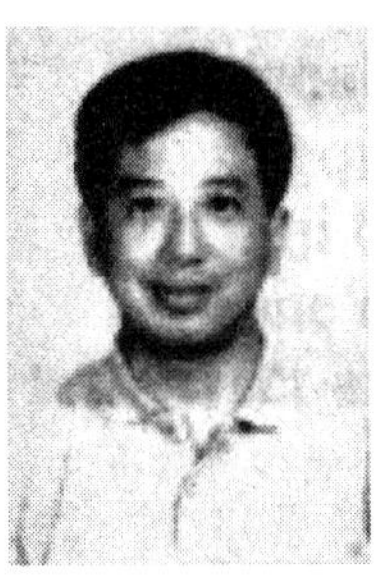

Dr. Chen Ken graduated from the Department of Traditional Chinese Medicine of the Anhui Medical College in 1976. From 1979 to 1981, he pursued post-graduate studies in the same department of the Beijing College of Traditional Chinese Medicine. In 1987, he was invited to Sweden and Finland to teach acupuncture. He is now teaching at the Beijing University of Traditional Chinese Medicine.

1. In recent years, he has been invited for several times to Europe to teach, supervise clinic, attend conferences and organize examinations. He is now managing a TCM Tele-consultation & services system for foreign practitioners of TCM who seek academic relationship with top Chinese experts.

Part One Multiple-choice Questions

"A" Type Questions

These have a stem and four or five options, of which only ONE is correct.

Example:
From which point does the branch of the Lung channel of the Hand-Taiyin proximal to the forearm emerge? (B)

A: Kongzui (Lu 6)
B: Lieque (Lu 7)
C: Jingqu (Lu 8)
D: Yuji (Lu 10)
E: none of the above

The correct answer is B, and is filled in the ( ).

I. Yin-Yang and the Five Elements

1. According to the theory of yin-yang, all the following conditions belong to opposite aspects within the same phenomenon except ( ).

A: day and night
B: brightness and dimness
C: movement and stillness
D: heat and cold
E: upward and inward

2. The time belonging to yin within yin is ( ).

A: the morning
B: the afternoon
C: the first half of the night
D: the second half of the night

E: none of the above

3. The time belonging to yang within yin is ( ).

A: the morning
B: the afternnon
C: the first half of the night
D: the second half of the night
E: none of the above

4. Which one of the following belongs to yin within yang? ( )

A: the morning
B: the afternoon
C: the first half of the night
D: the second half of the night
E: none of the above

5. Which one of the following belongs to yang within yang? ( )

A: the morning
B: the afternoon
C: the first half of the night
D: the second half of the night
E: none of the above

6. The symbols of yin and yang are ( ).

A: cold and heat
B: water and fire
C: upward and downward
D: brightness and dimness
E: movement and stillness

7. Which of the following pathological factors belongs to yin? ( )

A: wind
B: heat
C: damp
D: summer heat
E: none of the above

8. The property of yang is ( ).

A: downward
B: inward
C: stillness
D: excitement

E: inhibition

9. Which of the following properties belongs to yin? ( )

A: inhibition
B: brightness
C: upward direction
D: outward direction
E: warming

10. All the following properties belong to yang except ( ).

A: excitement
B: moving
C: warming
D: brightness
E: nourishing

11. All the following properties belong to yin except ( ).

A: weakness
B: nourishing
C: moving
D:moistening
E: dimness

12. The part of the human body pertaining to yang is ( ).

A: the medial aspects of the four limbs
B: the lower limbs
C: the back
D: the abdomen
E: the chest

13. The part of the human body pertaining to yin is ( ).

A: the medial aspects of the lower limbs
B: the lateral aspects of the upper limbs
C: the back
D: the head
E: Fu organs

14. According to the basic theory of yin and yang, weakness of yang leading to insufficiency of yin is due to ( ).

A: the opposition of yin and yang
B: the interdependence of yin and yang
C: the inter-consuming-supporting relationship of yin and yang

D: the inter-transforming relationship of yin and yang
E: the infinite divisibility of yin and yang

15. According to the basic theory of yin and yang, a preponderance of yin damaging yang is due to ( ).

A: the interdependence of yin and yang
B: the opposition of yin and yang
C: the inter-consuming-supporting relationship of yin and yang
D: the inter-transforming relationship of yin and yang
E: the infinite divisibility of yin and yang

16. According to the classification of the Five Elements, which of the following channels belongs to the wood? ( )

A: Hand-shaoyin channel
B: Hand-Jueyin channel
C: Hand-Shaoyang channel
D: Foot-Jueyin channel
E: Foot-Taiyin channel

17. According to the classification of the Five Elements, which of the following tastes belongs to metal? ( )

A: sour
B: bitter
C: sweet
D: pungent
E: salty

18. All the following belong to water except ( ).

A: kidney
B: ear
C: north
D: black
E: skin

19. According to the theory of the Five Elements, all the following belong to fire except ( ).

A: small intestine
B: anger
C: vessels
D: joy
E: summer

20. Which of the following relationships belongs to "mother" and "son"? ( )

A: water and fire
B:earth and metal
C: metal and wood
D: wood and earth
E: metal and fire

21. According to the theory of the Five Elements, the liver fire attacking the lung belongs to ( ).

A: "mother" disease affecting "son"
B: "son" disease affecting "mother"
C: interacting
D:overacting
E: counteracting

22. Hyperactivity of the liver attacking the spleen belongs to ( ).

A: interacting
B:overacting
C: counteracting
D:"mother" disease affecting "son"
E: "son" disease affecting "son"

23. The liver disease transmitting to the kidney belong to ( ).

A:"the son affecting the mother"
B: "the mother affecting the son"
C: interacting
D:overacting
E: counteracting

24. According to the theory of the Five Elements, the kidney disease transmitting to the spleen belongs to ( ).

A: "the son affecrting the mother"
B: "the mother affecting the son"
C: interacting
D: overacting
E:counteracting

25. According to the theory of the Five Elements, the spleen disease transmitting to the liver belongs to ( ).

A: interacting
B: "the mother affecting the son"

C: "the son affecting the mother"
D: counteracting
E: overacting

26. Which of the following methods follows the law of interacting of the Five Elements? ( )

A: strengthening the earth to produce metal
B: nourishing the water to nourish the wood
C: reinforcing the fire to tonify the earth
D: strengthening the metal to control the wood
E: none of the above

27. All the following methods follow the law of inter-promoting of the Five Elements except ( ).

A: strengthening the earth to produce the metal
B: strengthening the earth to control the wood
C: reinforcing the metal and water mutually
D: reinforcing the fire to tonify the earth
E: nourishing the water to nourish the wood

28. According to the Five-Shu points corresponding to the Five Elements, which o f the following points belongs to the metal? ( )

A: Zuqiaoyi (G 44)
B: Erjian (LI 2)
C: Shaoshang (L 11)
D: Taiyuan (L 9)
E: Xiangu (S 43)

29. According to the principle of reinforcing the "mother point" for deficiency syndrome, which of the following points would you select to treat the deficiency of the liver? ( )

A: Taichong (Liv 3)
B: Yingu (K 10)
C: Zhongfeng (Liv 4)
D: Taixi (K 3)
E: Rangu (K 2)

30. According to the principle of reducing the "son point" for excess syndrome , which of the following points would you select to treat the excess syndrome of the heart? ( )

A: Shaohai (H 3)

B: Lingdao (H 4)
C: Shenmen (H 7)
D: Shaofu (H 8)
E: Shaochong (H 9)

II. Zang-Fu, Qi, Blood and Body Fluid

1. All the following are Zang organs except the ( ).
A: heart
B: kidney
C: bladder
D: spleen
E: liver

2. All the following are Fu organs except the ( ).
A: small intestine
B: large intestine
C: Sanjiao
D: lung
E: stomach

3. All the following are extraordinary Fu organs except the ( ).
A: brain
B: pericardium
C: gallbladder
D: bones
E: uterus

4. Which of the following is considered both Fu and extraordinary Fu organ? ( )
A: uterus
B: vessels
C: Sanjiao
D: bladder
E: gallbladder

5. Which of the following organs has the function of housing the mind? ( )
A: heart
B: lung

C: liver
D: kidney
E: brain

6. Which of the following organs has the function of storing blood? (　)

A: heart
B: liver
C: kidney
D: pericardium
E: none of the above

7. The heart is the (　).

A: house for storing the blood
B: source for production of the blood
C: motive force for blood circulation
D: sea of blood
E: none of the above

8. Which of the following sense organs is connected with the heart? (　)

A: eye
B: tongue
C: mouth
D: nose
E: ear

9. Which of the following Fu organs has an interior-exterior relationship to the heart? (　)

A: stomach
B: bladder
C: gallbladder
D: small intestine
E: large intestine

10. The liver (　).

A: produces the blood
B: regulates the volume of the blood in circulation
C: is the primary organ in charge of blood circulation
D: controls the blood by keeping it within the vessels
E: none of the above

11. Where does the blood store during sleep? (　)

A: in the heart

B: in the spleen
C: in the liver
D: in the kidney
E: in the brain

12. Which of the following sense organs is connected to the liver? (   )

A: eye
B:tongue
C: mouth
D: nose
E: ear

13. Which of the following Fu organs has an interior-exterior relationship with the liver? (   )

A: stomach
B: bladder
C: gallbladder
D: small intestine
E: Sanjiao

14. The liver controls (   ).

A: vessels
B: bones
C: muscles
D: tendons
E: four limbs

15. Which of the following effects the function of the liver in maintaining the free flow of Qi? (   )

A: emotional activity
B: ascending and descending function of the stomach and spleen
C: secretion of bile
D: all of the above (include A, B and C)
E: none of the above.

16. Which of the following physiological phenomenon is not closely linked with the function of the liver for maintaining the free flow of Qi? (   )

A: movement of Qi
B: circulation of blood
C: digestion
D: contraction and relaxation of the tendons and muscles

E: emotional activity

17. Which of the following organs has a close relationship with the condition of the nail? ( )

A: liver
B: heart
C: kidney
D: lung
E: spleen

18. Which of the following organs has the property of keeping the blood circulating within the vessels and preventing extravasation? ( )

A: heart
B: liver
C: spleen
D: lung
E: kidney

19. The condition of the spleen is manifested on the ( ).

A: lips
B: nails
C: hair
D: skin
E: ear

20. A normal sense of taste is linked with the function of the ( ).

A: liver
B: spleen
C: lung
D: heart
E: kidney

21. The digestion, absorption and transmission of nutrients are the function of the ( ).

A: spleen
B: stomach
C: liver
D: kidney
E: small intestine

22. In TCM which of the following Zang organs is most superficial? ( )

A: heart

B: lung
C: spleen
D: liver
E: kidney

23. In TCM the sense of smell depends on the ( ).
A: spleen
B: heart
C: lung
D: liver
E: kidney

24. Which of the following organs regulates water passage? ( )
A: spleen
B: lung
C: liver
D: bladder
E: gallbladder

25. The distribution of defensive Qi (Wei Qi) depends on the function of ( ).
A: heart
B: lung
C: liver
D: kidney
E: spleen

26. The opening and closing of the pores are dominated by the ( ).
A: kidney
B: liver
C: spleen
D: heart
E: lung

27. Which of the following organs has the function of storing essence? ( )
A: heart
B: lung
C: liver
D: spleen
E: kidney

28. The acquired essence is produced and transformed by the ( ).
A: lung and large intestine

B: heart and small intestine
C: kidney and bladder
D: liver and gallbladder
E: spleen and stomach

29. The acquired essence is stored in (   ).

A: heart
B: spleen
C: liver
D: kidney
E: lung

30. Which of the following organs is said to be "the house of the water and fire"? (   )

A: heart
B: liver
C: kidney
D: lung
E: spleen

31. Which of the following organs dominates the development and reproduction? ( )

A: heart
B: kidney
C: spleen
D: liver
E: lung

32. Which of the following organs dominates the water metabolism? (   )

A: spleen
B: lung
C: kidney
D: bladder
E: heart

33. Which of the following organs dominates the urethra and genitals? (   )

A: liver
B: kidney
C: spleen
D: large intestine
E: bladder

34. The ear relates to ( ).

A: heart
B: liver
C: spleen
D: kidney
E:lung

35. Deficiency of the kidney Qi may cause ( ).

A: enuresis
B: anuria
C: diarrhoea
D: constipation
E: all of them mentioned above

36. Which of the following relates to the bone? ( )

A: nail
B: hair
C: teeth
D: tendon
E: muscle

37. The bones are dominated by ( ).

A: kidney
B: liver
C: spleen
D: heart
E: lung

38. The brain is considered the sea of ( ).

A: Qi
B: blood
C: nutrient substance
D: marrow
E: body fluid

39. The condition of the kidney is manifested on ( ).

A: skin
B: hair
C: face
D: nail
E: lips

40. Which of the following organ pairs is known as the source of the "acquired foundation"? ( )

A: spleen and stomach
B: lung and large intesitine
C: kidney and bladder
D: liver and gallbladder
E: heart and small intestine

41. The kidney receiving Qi means ( ).

A: the kidney assists the lung in its function of receiving and helping the Qi to decend
B: the kidney is the place for the storage of essential Qi
C: the kidney is the place for producing essential Qi
D: the kidney dominates water metabolism
E: the kidney promotes the function of the lung dispersing Qi

42. The kidney has the function of ( ).

A: dominating Qi
B: producing Qi
C: receiving Qi
D: regulating Qi
E: transporting Qi

43. The uterus is connected with the following organs and channels except ( ).

A: the kidney channel
B: the Chong channel
C: the liver channel
D: the lung channel
E: the Ren channel

44. The Qi stored in the chest which can promote the functions of the lung and heart is called ( ).

A: Yuanqi (Primary Qi)
B: Zongqi (Pectoral Qi)
C: Yingqi (Nutrient Qi)
D: Weiqi (Defensive Qi)
E: none of the above

45. The body fluid has the function of ( ).

A: promoting

B: warming
C: protecitng
D:checking
E:nourishing

46 The Qi circulating within the vessels which can transform into blood is called ( ).

A: Yuanqi (Primary Qi)
B: Zongqi (Pectoral Qi)
C: Yingqi (Nutrient Qi)
D: Weiqi (Defensive Qi)
E: Xinqi (Heart Qi)

III. The Channels, Collaterals and Acupoints

1. Where do the yang channels of the hands meet the yang channels of the feet? ( )

A: forehead
B: face
C: upper limbs
D: chest and abdomen
E: lower limbs

2. Where do the three yin channels of the hand meet the three yin channels of the foot? ( )

A: head
B: face
C: chest
D: abdomen
E: limbs

3. Where do the yin channels and the yang channels which have an interior exterior relationship meet? ( )

A: head
B: face
C: chest
D: abdomen
E: four limbs

4. The lung channel originates from the ( ).

A: lung
B: upper jiao
C: middle jiao
D: lower jiao
E: chest

5. Which of the following channels originates in the middle jiao? ( )

A: Ren chennel
B: Du channel
C: Chong channel
D: lung channel
E: heart channel

6. The pathway of the Hand-Yangming channel does not pass through ( ).

A: the forearms
B: the upperarms
C: the radial side of the index finger
D: the medial side of the elbow
E: the neck

7. The tibial branch of the stomach channel emerges from ( ).

A: Zusanli (S 36)
B: Shangjuxu (S 37)
C: Tiaokou (S 38)
D: Xiajuxu (S 39)
E: Fenglong (S 40)

8. The branch of the stomach channel from the dorsum of the foot arises from ( ) .

A: Jiexi (S 41)
B: Chongyang (S 42)
C: Xiangu (S 43)
D: Neiting (S 44)
E: Lidui (S 45)

9. The tibial branch of the stomach channel terminates at ( ).

A: the medial side of the big toe
B: the lateral side of the big toe
C: the lateral side of the middle toe
D: the medial side of the middle toe

E: none of the above

10. The dorsum of the foot branch of the stomach channel terminates at ( ).

A: the medial side of the big toe
B: the lateral side of the big toe
C: the lateral side of the middle toe
D: the medial side of the middle toe
E: none of the above

11. All the following organs are linked with the kidney channel except ( ).

A: the liver
B: the heart
C: the spleen
D: the lung
E: the kidney

12. The branch of the lung channel proximal to the wrist emerges from ( ).

A: Kongzui (L 6)
B: Lieque (L 7)
C: Jingqu (L 8)
D: Taiyuan (L 9)
E: Yuji (L 10)

13. The channel entering the ear is ( ).

A: the Hand-Yangming channel
B: the Foot-Yangming channel
C: the Foot-Taiyang channel
D: the Hand-Taiyang Channel
E: none of the above

14. Which of the following channels has a branch which arises from the lung, joins the heart and runs into the chest? ( )

A: Hand-Taiyin
B: Foot-Shaoyin
C: Hand-Taiyang
D: Foot-Taiyin
E: Hand-Shaoyin

15. All the following channels pass through the lung except ( ).

A: Hand-Jueyin
B: Hand-Shaoyin
C: Foot-Jueyin

D: Foot-Shaoyin
E: Hand-Yangming

16. The branch of the pericardium channel which links with the Sanjiao channel a rises from ( ).

A: Ximen (P 4)
B: Jianshi (P 5)
C: Neiguan (P 6)
D: Daling (P 7)
E: Laogong (P 8)

17. The branch of the gallbladder channel from the dorsum of the foot arises from ( ).

A: Qiuxu (G 40)
B: Foot-Linqi (G 41)
C: Diwuhui (G 42)
D: Xiaxi (G 43)
E: none of the above

18. The branch of the gallbladder channel from the dorsum of the foot terminates at ( ).

A: the medial side of the big toe
B: the lateral side of the big toe
C: the hairy region of the big toe
D: the lateral side of the fourth toe
E: the medial side of the fourth toe

19. Which of the following channels has a branch which arises from the retroauricular region, enters the ear, then exits and passes through the preauricular region? ( )

A: Foot-Shaoyang
B: Foot-Taiyin
C: Hand-Taiyang
D: Foot-Jueyin
E: Hand-Yangming

20. Which of the following channels does not run superiorly towards the head and face? ( )

A: heart channel
B: liver channel
C: Chong channel

D: Yinwei channel
E: Yinqiao channel

21. On the abdomen, the Chong channel communicates with ( ).
A: the Ren channel
B: the stomach channel
C: the kidney channel
D: the spleen channel
E: none of the above

22. On the abdomen, the Yinwei channel communicates with ( ).
A: the spleen channel
B: the stomach channel
C: the kidney channel
D: the Ren channel
E: none of the above

23. At the neck, the Yinwei channel communicates with ( ).
A: the Ren channel
B: the stomach channel
C: the large intestine channel
E: the small intestine channel
E: none of the above

24. The distance between the two mastoid processes is ( ).
A: 6 cun
B: 8 cun
C: 9 cun
D: 10 cun
E: 12 cun

25. The distance between the two nipples is ( ).
A: 5 cun
B: 6 cun
C: 8 cun
D: 9 cun
E: 10 cun

26. The distance from the anterior hairline to the posterior hairline is ( ).
A: 8 cun
B: 9 cun
C: 10 cun

D: 12 cun
E: 13 cun

27. The distance from the sternocostal angle to the centre of the umbilicus is ( ).

A: 8 cun
B: 9 cun
C: 10 cun
D: 12 cun
E: 13 cun

28. The distance between the medial border of the scapula and the posterior midline is ( ).

A: 2 cun
B: 3 cun
C: 4 cun
D: 5 cun
E: 6 cun

29. The distance between the end of the axillary fold and the transverse cubital crease is ( ).

A: 6 cun
B: 7 cun
C: 8 cun
D: 9 cun
E: 10 cun

30. The distance between the transverse cubital crease and the transverse wrist crease is ( ).

A: 8 cun
B: 9 cun
C: 10 cun
D: 12 cun
E: 13 cun

31. The distance between the superior border of the symphysis pubis and the medial epicondyle of the femur is ( ).

A: 12 cun
B: 10 cun
C: 13 cun
D: 16 cun

E: 18 cun

32. The distance between the inferior border of the medial condyle of the tibia and the tip of the medial malleolus is ( ).

A: 8 cun
B: 10 cun
C: 12 cun
D: 13 cun
E: 16 cun

33. The distance between the prominence of the trochanter and the middle of the patella is ( ).

A: 16 cun
B: 18 cun
C: 19 cun
D: 20 cun
E: 22 cun

34. The distance between the centre of the patella and the tip of the lateral malleolus is ( ).

A: 16 cun
B: 18 cun
C: 19 cun
D: 20 cun
E: 22 cun

35. The distance between the tip of the lateral malleolus and the heel is ( ).

A: 1 cun
B: 2 cun
C: 3 cun
D: 4 cun
E: 6 cun

36. The distance between the centre of the umbilicus and the superior border of the symphysis pubis is ( ).

A: 3 cun
B: 4 cun
C: 5 cun
D: 6 cun
E: 8 cun

37. The distance between the end of the axillary fold on the lateral side of the chest and the tip of the eleventh rib is ( ).

A: 8 cun
B: 9 cun
C: 10 cun
D: 12 cun
E: 13 cun

38. The distance between Yintang (Extra) and Baihui (Du 20) is ( ).

A: 18 cun
B: 15 cun
C: 8 cun
D: 12 cun
E: 10 cun

39. The distance between Guanyuan (Ren 4) and Jiuwei (Ren 15) is ( ).

A: 8 cun
B: 9 cun
C: 5 cun
D: 13 cun
E: 10 cun

40. The distance between the following pair of points is 1.5 cun except ( ).

A: Qihai (Ren 6)-Shenjue (Ren 8)
B: Neiguan (P 6)-Daling (P 7)
C: Shenmen (H 7)-Lingdao (H 4)
D: Xinshu (B 15)-Shentang (B 44)
E: Dushu (B 16)-Lingtai (Du 10)

41. The distance between the following pair of points is 0.5 cun except ( ).

A: Yamen (Du 15)-Fengfu (Du 16)
B: Yinxi (H 6)-Shenmen (H 7)
C: Jingqu (L 8)-Taiyuan (L 9)
D: Shimen (Ren 5)-Qihai (Ren 6)
E: Qihai (Ren-6)-Yinjiao (Ren 7)

42. The distance between the following pair of points is 3 cun except ( ).

A: Fuyang (B 59)-Kunlun (B 60)
B: Dubi (S 35)-Zusanli (S 36)
C: Ligou (Liv 5)-Zhongdu (Liv 6)
D: Futu (S 32)-Yinshi (S 33)
E: Yangxi (LI 5)-Pianli (LI 6)

43. Which of the following pair of points is 2 cun apart? ( )

A: Waiguan (SJ 5)-Sanyangluo (SJ 8)
B: Xialian (LI 8)-Shanglian (LI 9)
C: Yangxi (LI 5)-Pianli (LI 6)
D: Daling (P 7)-Jianshi (P 5)
E: none of the above

44. Which of the following pair of points is 8 cun apart? ( )

A: Taiyuan (L 9)-Kongzui (L 6)
B: Pianli (LI 6)-Quchi (LI 11)
C: Zusanli (S 36)-Fenglong (S 40)
D: Sanyinjiao (Sp 6)-Yinlingquan (P 9)
E: Zhongji (Ren 3)-Zhongwan (Ren 12)

45. All the following points are located 3 cun above the transverse crease of the wrist except ( ).

A: Pianli (LI 6)
B: Zhizheng (SI 7)
C: Zhigou (SJ 6)
D: Huizong (SJ 7)
E: Jianshi (P 5)

46. When the index finger and thumbs of both hands are crossed with the index finger of one hand placed on the styloid process of the radius of the other, the depression right under the tip of the index finger is ( ).

A: Jingqu (L 8)
B: Lieque (L 7)
C: Yangxi (LI 5)
D: Pianli (LI 6)
E: none of the above

47. Lieque (L 7) is a/an ( ).

A: Xi-Cleft point
B: Luo-Connecting point
C: Jing-River point
D: influential point
E: none of the above

48. Which of the following points is most likely to be selected to treat neck rigidity? ( )

A: Zhongfu (L 1)

B: Chize (L 5)
C: Lieque (L 7)
D: Taiyuan (L 9)
E: Yuji (L 10)

49. Taiyuan (L 9) is a/an ( ).
A: Shu-Stream point
B: Yuan-Source point
C: influential point of the channels
D: earth point on the lung channel
E: all of the above

50. The three yin channels of the hand are commonly indicated in ( ).
A: mental illness
B: disorders of the heart
C: disorders of the stomach
D: disorders of the chest
E: none of the above

51. The three yang channels of the hand are commonly indicated in ( ).
A: disorders of the forehead, face and nose
B: disorders of the mouth and teeth
C: disorders of the eye, throat and febrile diseases
D: disorders of the ear
E: none of the above

52. Which of the following points is located 2 cun below Quchi (LI 11)? ( )
A: Pianli (LI 6)
B: Wenliu (LI 7)
C: Xialian (LI 8)
D: Shanglian (LI 9)
E: Shousanli (LI 10)

53. All the following points are on the line joining Yangxi (LI 5) and Quchi (LI 11) except ( ).
A: Wenliu (LI 7)
B: Shousanli (LI 10)
C: Zhouliao (LI 12)
D: Xialian (LI 8)
E: Pianli (LI 6)

54. Wenliu (LI 7) is a (   ).

A: Luo-Connecting point
B: Jing-River point
C: Yuan-Source point
D: Xi-Cleft point
E: none of the above

55. Which of the following points is level with the tip of Adam's apple, on the anterior border of m. sternocleidomastoideus? (   )

A: Futu (LI 18)
B: Daying (S 5)
C: Renying (S 9)
D: Shuitu (S 10)
E: Lianquan (Ren 23)

56. Which of the following points is located 1 cun above the umbilicus, and 2 cun lateral to Shuifen (Ren 9)? (   )

A: Burong (S 19)
B: Guanmen (S 22)
C: Taiyi (S 23)
D: Chengman (S 20)
E: Huaroumen (S 24)

57. Which of the following points is the most commonly used for clearing the stomach heat? (   )

A: Weishu (B 21)
B: Neiting (S 44)
C: Fenglong (S 40)
D: Chongyang (S 42)
E: Liangqiu (S 34)

58. Which of the following groups of points is level with Jianli (Ren 11)? (   )

A: Guanmen (S 22) and Shiguan (K 18)
B: Liangmen (S 21) and Youmen (K 21)
C: Chengman (S 20) and Siman (K 14)
D: Taiyi (S 23) and Shangqu (K 17)
E: Burong (S 19) and Abdomen-Tonggu (K 20)

59. Which of the following points is level with Chengman (S 20)? (   )

A: Jujue (Ren 14)
B: Jiuwei (Ren 15)

C: Youmen (K 21)
D: Abdomen-Tonggu (K 20)
E: Bulang (K 22)

60. The point on the line 4 cun below the umbilicus is ( ).

A: Henggu (K 11)
B: Dahe (K 12)
C: Daju (S 27)
D: Shuidao (S 28)
E: Qixue (K 13)

61. The point which is in the depression distal and inferior to the base of the first matatarsal bone is ( ).

A: Dadu (Sp 2)
B: Taibai (Sp 3)
C: Gongsun (Sp 4)
D: Taichong (Liv 3)
E: Zhongfeng (Liv 4)

62. Which of the following points can be used with Gongsun (Sp 4) to treat disorders of the stomach, heart and chest? ( )

A: Zusanli (S 36)
B: Zhongwan (Ren 12)
C: Neiguan (P 6)
D: Shenmen (H 7)
E: Shanzhong/Tanzhong (Ren 17)

63. Which of the following points would you select for the treatment of difficult labour? ( )

A: Zhongchong (P 9)
B: Zuqiaoyin (G 44)
C: Zhiyin (B 67)
D: Lidui (S 45)
E: Shaochong (H 9)

64. Which of the following points would you select for the treatment of malposion? ( )

A: Zhongchong (P 9)
B: Foot-Qiaoyin (G 44)
C: Zhiyin (B 67)
D: Lidui (S 45)

E: Shaochong (H 9)

65. Which of the following points is often used to treat insufficient lactation? ( )

A: Shaoze (SI 1)
B: Shaochong (H 9)
C: Zhongchong (P 9)
D: Lidui (S 45)
E: Yinbai (Sp 1)

66. The point with the function of strengthening the spleen, soothing the liver and tonifying the kidney is ( ).

A: Yinlingquan (Sp 9)
B: Sanyinjiao (Sp 6)
C: Pishu (B 20)
D: Zusanli (S 36)
E: Guanyuan (Ren 4)

67. The point located in the centre of the suprascapular fossa is ( ).

A: Bingfeng (SI 12)
B: Tianzong (SI 11)
C: Jianwaishu (SI 14)
D: Naoshu (SI 10)
E: Quyuan (SI 13)

68. The point located level with Dazhui (Du 14) is ( ).

A: Jianwaishu (SI 14)
B: Jianzhongshu (SI 15)
C: Quyuan (SI 13)
D: Dazhu (B 11)
E: none of the above

69. The point most commonly used in the treatment of various blood syndromes is ( ).

A: Shenmen (H 7)
B: Weizhong (B 40)
C: Taibai (Sp 3)
D: Geshu (B 17)
E: Xinshu (B 15)

70. The point which has the function of dispersing wind, removing heat and benefiting eyes is ( ).

A: Jingming (UB 1)

B: Quchi (LI 11)
C: Yifeng (SJ 17)
D: Shangxing (DU 23)
E: Fengchi (G 20)

71. Which of the following channels has the most branches? (   )
A: bladder channel
B: stomach channel
C: gallbladder channel
D: liver channel
E: Sanjiao channel

72. Which channel originates from the nose? (   )
A: stomach channel
B: spleen channel
C: bladder channel
D: gallbladder channel
E: none of the above

73. What point is located between the bilateral Ganshu (B 17)? (   )
A: Jingsuo (Du 8)
B: Zhongshu (Du 7)
C: Xuanshu (Du 5)
D: Zhiyang (Du 9)
E: none of the above

74. The therapeutic effect of combining Hegu (LI 4) and Fengchi (G 20) is (   ).
A: clearing heat and detoxifying
B: dispersing superficial pathogenic wind
C: mediating the Shaoyang channel
D: relieving cough and asthma
E: subduing hyperactivity of the yang of the liver

75. Hegu (LI 4) has the effect of regulating sweating as does the point (   ).
A: Dazhui (Du 14)
B: Taodao (Du 13)
C: Taixi (K 3)
D: Fuliu (K 7)
E: Pianli (LI 6)

76. The points Shaofu (H 8) and Laogong (P 8) are commonly used together to ( ).

A: house the mind
B: clear the fire of the heart
C: regulate the Qi of the liver
D: cure night sweating
E: dredge the channels and collaterals

77. Which of the following points has the property of regulating the heart rate? ( )

A: Zusanli (S 36)
B: Neiguan (P 6)
C: Hegu (LI 4)
D: Juque (Ren 14)
E: Shenmen (H 7)

78. Which of the following points is the most appropriate to treat hernia? ( )

A: Yongquan (K 1)
B: Yinbai (Sp 1)
C: Dadun (Liv 1)
D: Foot-Qiaoyin (G 44)
E: Zhiyin (B 67)

79. What action would it produce when the Lianquan (Ren 23) and Zhaohai (K 6) are stimulated simultaneously? ( )

A: relieving anxiety
B: promoting circulation of blood and Qi and relaxing muscles and tendons
C: subduing endogenous wind and relieving phlegm
D: regulating the function of the stomach to stop vomitting
E: promoting secretion of body fluid to relieve thirst

80. There is no Front-Mu point located on the pathway of ( ).

A: the lung channel
B: the spleen channel
C: the liver channel
D: the gallbladder channel
E: the Ren channel

81. The point level with Xiawan (Ren 10) is ( ).

A. Liangmen (S 21)
B: Taiyi (S 23)

C: Daheng (SP 15)
D:Dahe (K 12)
E: Shuidao (S 28)

82. Renying (S 9) is ( ) cun lateral to Adam's apple.

A: 1.5
B: 2
C: 2.5
D: 3
E: 3.5

83. Which of the following points is located 2 cun above the laterosuperior bord er of the patella? ( )

A: Xuehai (SP 10)
B: Zusanli (S 36)
C: Liangqiu (S 34)
D: Futu (S 32)
E: Fengshi (G 31)

84. Which of the following points is stimulated when dealing with sore throat? ( )

A: Shaochong (H 9)
B: Zhongchong (P 9)
C: Shaoshang (L 11)
D: Shaoze (SI 1)
E: Yongquan (K 1)

85. The most effective point in reducing a high-grade fever would be ( ).

A: Jianjing (G 21)
B: Fengfu (Du 17)
C: Renzhong (Du 26)
D: Quchi (LI 11)
E: Yamen (Du 15)

86. The channel/channels with the function of regulating the movements of the extremities as well as the opening and closing of the eyelids is/are ( ).

A: Du channel
B: bladder channel
C: gallbladder channel
D: Yinqiao and Yangqiao channels
E: Yinwei and Yangwei channels

87. Which of the following channels has influential points that are frequently employed to treat insomnia? ( )

A: Yinwei channel
B: Yangwei channel
C: Chong channel
D: Yinqiao channel
E: Yangqiao channel

88. Which of the following extraordinary channels has influential points that are often selected in dealing with somnolence? ( )

A: Yinwei channel
B: Yangwei channel
C: Chong channel
D: Yinqiao channel
E: Yangqiao channel

89. All the following specific points are located below the elbow joints or knee joints except ( ).

A: the eight confluent points
B: the Five-Shu points
C: the Luo-Connecting points of the 12 regular channels
D: the eight influential points
E: the Yuan-Source points

90. When a patient is standing erect with his hands hanging down at his sides, what point do the tips of the middle fingers touch? ( )

A: Zhongdu (G 32)
B: Xiyangguan (G 33)
C: Fengshi (G 31)
D: Juliao (G 29)
E: Yanglingquan (G 34)

91. The point midway between Dazhui (Du 14) and the acromion is ( ).

A: Quyuan (SI 13)
B: Tianliao (SJ 15)
C: Jianjing (G 21)
D: Jugu (LI 16)
E: Bingfeng (SI 12)

92. Which of the following statements is correct? ( )

A: Ligou (Liv 5) is a Xi-Cleft point

B: Foot-Zhongdu (Liv 6) is a Jing-River point
C: Zhongfeng (Liv 4) is a Luo-Connecting point
D: Xiguan (Liv 7) is a He-Sea point
E: none of the above

93. The function of Tanzhong (Ren 17) is ( ).
A: smoothing the chest and regulating Qi.
B: strengthening the spleen and eliminating phlegm
C: harmonizing the stomach
D: tranquilizing the liver
E: moving blood

94. Sanyinjiao (SP 6) is ( ).
A: a He-Sea point
B: a Yuan-Source point
C: a Luo-Connecting point
D: a confluent point
E: none of the above

95. The points of the gallbladder channel on the posteiror border of the fibula are ( ).
A: Waiqiu (G 36) and Yangfu (G 38)
B: Yangjiao (G 35) and Xuanzhong (G 39)
C: Guangming (G 37) and Yanglingquan (G 34)
D: Qiuxu (G 40) and Foot-Linqi (G 41)
E: none of the above

96. Yangjiao (G 35) is ( ).
A: a Xi-Cleft point
B: one of the eight confluent points
C: one of the eight influential points
D: a Jing-River point
E: none of the above

97. The twelve regular channels are named after ( ).
A: Yin-Yang, the Five Elements and Zang-Fu organs
B: Hand-foot, the Five elements and Zang-Fu organs
C: the Five Elements, hand-foot and Zang-Fu organs
D: Zang-Fu organs, hand-foot and yin-yang
E: Zang-Fu organs, hand-foot and the Five Elements

98. The channel which abound in blood and have relatively less Qi is (   ).

A: Yangming and Taiyang channels
B: Taiyang and Jueyin channels
C: Shaoyang and Shaoyin channels
D: Taiyin and Shaoyang channels
E: none of the above

99. The point between the tendons of m.semitendinosus and semimembranosus (when the knee is flexed) is (   ).

A: Yingu (K 10)
B: Yanggu (SI 5)
C: Ququan (Liv 8)
D: Weizhong (UB 40)
E: Weiyang (UB 39)

100. A point frequently selected in treating blood diseases is (   ).

A: Guanyuan (Ren 4)
B: Qihai (Ren 6)
C: Geshu (UB 17)
D: Weizhong (UB 40)
E: Gaohuangshu (UB 43)

101. A prescription containing the points Dazhui (Du 14), Fengmen (UB 12) and Shaoshang (Lu 11) has an action of (   ).

A: tonifying the yin of the lung
B: activating the dispersing function of the lung to relieve the exterior symptoms
C: eliminating wind and soothing asthma
D: activating the function of the stomach and the spleen
E: none of the above

102. The pathway of the Chong channel on the abdomen coincides with that of (   ).

A: the Ren channel
B: the stomach channel
C: the kidney channel
D: the spleen channel
E: none of the above

103. Which of the following statements about the Chong channel is incorrect? (   )

A: It is the “sea” of blood

B: It is the "sea" of the twelve regular organs
C: It is the "sea" of Qi
D: It is the "sea" of the five Zang and six Fu
E: All of the above are correct

104. Which of the following statements about the Jing-Well points in light of the theory of Yin-Yang and the Five Elements is correct ( ).

A: The Jing-Well point on Yang channel is attributed to metal and the Jing-Well point on Yin channel is attributed to wood.
B: The Jing-Well point on Yang channel is attributed to water and the Jing-Well point on Yin channel is attributed to fire.
C: The Jing-Well point on Yang channel is attributed to wood and the Jing-Well point on Yin channel is attributed to earth.
D: The Jing-Well point on Yang channel is attributed to fire and the Jing-Well point on Yin channel is attributed to metal.
E: The Jing-Well point on Yang channel is attributed to earth and the Jing-Well point on Yin channel is attributed to water.

105. Each of the following channels passes the lung (organ) except ( ).

A: the Hand-Jueying channel
B: the Hand-Shaoyang channel
C: the Foot-Jueying channel
D: the Foot-Shaoying channel
E. the Hand-Yangming channel

106. Which of the following points is remarkable in its ability to invigorate the spleen, tonify kidney-yin and nourish the blood? ( )

A: Taixi (K 3)
B:Guanyuan (Ren 4)
C: Sanyinjiao (Sp 6)
D: Zusanli (St 36)
E: Zhaohai (K 6)

107. Each of the following points is marked out in Fig. 1 except ( ).

A: Zhongchong (P 9)
B: Daling (P 7)

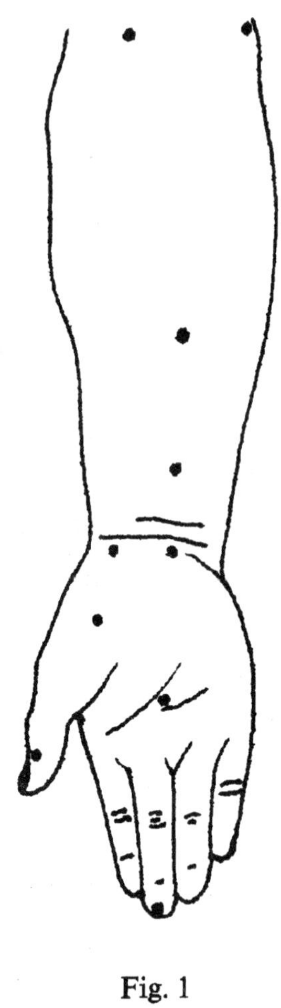

Fig. 1

C: Laogong (P 8)
D: Lieque (Lu 7)
E: Neiguan (P 6)

108. The points on the Ren and Du channels would exert similar therapeutic effectiveness in treating ( ).

A. febrile diseases
B: disorders of the face
C: lumbar back disorders
D: mental disorders
E: disorders of the throat

109. The reason Yin channel points treat disorders of the head is that ( ).

A: there is a close relationship between internal and external related organs
B: the collateral connects the Yin channels with the head
C: some points on the Yin channels have special functions
D: there is a close relationship between the divergent channels (Jingbie) and the twelve regular channels
E: the Yin and Yang channels are related through the Du and Ren channels

110. The circulation of the twelve regular channels includes each of the following except ( ).

A: the gallbladder channel—liver channel—lung channel
B: the large intestine channel—stomach channel—spleen channel
C: the heart channel—small intestine channel—urinary bladder channel
D: the kidney channel—small intestine channel—Sanjiao channel
E: the Sanjiao channel—gallbladder channel—liver channel

111. The order of the channels distributed to the abdomen, from the Ren channel to the exterior, are ( ).

A: Ren channel—spleen channel—kidney channel—stomach channel
B: Ren channel—kidney channel—spleen channel—stomach channel
C: Ren channel—stomach channel—spleen channel—kidney channel
D: Ren Channel—stomach channel—kidney channel—spleen channel
E: Ren channel—kidney channel—stomach channel—spleen channel

112. Each of the following organs has a connection to the course of the kidney channel except ( ).

A: the liver
B: the heart
C: the spleen

D: the lung
E: the kidney

113. The channels connecting with either the external or internal canthus include each of the following except ( ).

A: the Taiyang lung channel
B: the Shaoyang Sanjiao channel
C: the Yangming large intestine channel
D: the yangming stomach channel
E: the Shaoyang gallbladder channel

114. What is the total number of Front-Mu point on the body (bilateral point are counted as two points)? ( )

A: 12
B: 15
C: 18
D: 21
E: 24

115. All the following points are located distal to the elbow or knee joint except ( ).

A: the eight confluent points
B: the Five-Shu points
C: the Luo-connecting points
D: the eight influential points
E: the Yuan-Source points

116. Which is the most likely order the acupuncture points were discovered? ( )

A: points of the14 channels—extraordinary points—Ahshi points
B: extraordinary points—Ahshi points—points of the 14 channels
C: Ahshi points—points of the 14 channels—extraordinary points
D: Ahshi points—extraordinary points—points of the 14 channels
E: points of the 14 channels—Ahshi points—extraordinary points

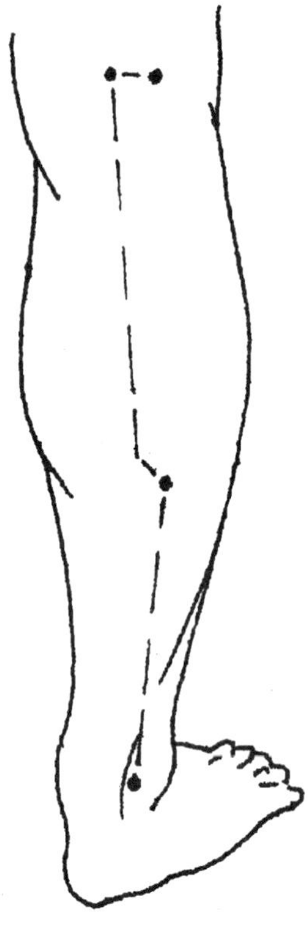

Fig. 2

117. The point which is not marked out in Fig. 2 would be ( ).

A: Kunlun (UB 60)

B: Feiyang (UB 58)
C: Weiyang (UB 39)
D: Weizhong (UB 40)
E: Chengshan (UB 57)

IV. Diagnostic Methods

1. A patient usually exhibits a pale complexion with all of the following syndromes except (   ).

A: deficiency of Qi
B: deficiency of blood
C: deficiency of yang
D: deficiency of yin
E: cold

2. The presence of malar flush indicates (   ).

A: damp heat in the liver and gallbladder
B: yin deficiency
C: Qi deficiency
D: deficiency of liver blood
E: invasion of pathologic heat

3. A dull (not bright) pale yellow complexion is a sign of (   ).

A: heart fire
B: invasion of pathologic heat
C: deficiency of both Qi and blood
D: deficiency of yang
E: deficiency of yin

4. A bluish complexion may be present in all of the following conditions except (   ).

A: cold syndromes
B: painful syndromes
C: stagnation of blood
D: retention of dampness
E: convulsions

5. Blue-purplish complexion and lips with the intermittent pain in the precordial region is due to (   ).

A: stagnation of heart blood

B: heat in the blood
C: deficiency of liver yin
D: attack of the heart by phlegm
E: deficiency of heart yin

6. A dark complexion (without brightness) accompanied by scaly skin indicates ( ).

A: deficiency of Qi
B: deficiency of yang
C: invasion of wind
D: invasion of cold
E: stagnation of blood

7. A swollen pale tongue with tooth prints on the border indicates ( ).

A: deficiency of heart Qi
B: deficiency of spleen and kidney yang
C: deficiency of the lung
D: deficiency of liver blood
E: deficiency of kidney yin

8. A swollen tongue which is deep red in colour indicates ( ).

A: excessive heat in the heart and spleen
B: invasion of the lung by pathologic heat
C: damp-heat in the liver
D: dampness and phlegm in the lung
E: yin deficiency of the heart and liver

9. A thin and dry tongue which is deep red in colour indicates ( ).

A: yin and Qi deficiency
B: Qi and blood deficiency
C: hyperactivity of fire due to deficiency of yin
D: damp-heat syndrome
E: stagnation of blood

10. A thorny and red tongue indicates ( ).

A: deficiency of blood
B: deficiency of yin
C: stagnation of blood
D: pathologic heat in the interior
E: none of the above

11. A cracked and red tongue indicates (　).

A: deficiency of blood
B: excessive heat
C: deficiency of yang
D: deficiency of lung Qi
E: weakness of the spleen

12. A cracked and pale tongue indicates (　).

A: deficiency of blood
B: deficiency of liver yin
C: damp-heat syndrome
D: invasion of pathologic cold
E: stagnation of blood

13. Which of the following conditions may be present in a normal person? (　)

A: swollen tongue
B: thin tongue
C: thorny tongue
D: tooth prints on the border
E: cracked tongue

14. A yellow dry tongue coating usually indicates (　).

A: exterior heat syndrome
B: inteiror heat syndrome
C: damp-heat syndrome
D: deficient heat syndrome
E: yin deficiency

15. The presence of purplish spots on the tongue surface indicates (　).

A: deficiency of Qi
B: deficiency of yin
C: stagnation of Qi
D: stagnation of blood
E: accumulation of phlegm

16. A pale purplish and moist tongue indicates (　).

A: deficiency of yin and retention of dampness
B: stagnation of Qi
C: stagnation of blood due to heat
D: stagnation of blood due to cold

E: deficiency of both Qi and blood

17. The thorns on the tip of the tongue indicate ( ).

A: liver and gallbladder fire
B: stomach fire
C: heart fire
D: deficiency of stomach yin
E: deficiency of kidney yin

18. A yellow sticky tongue coating indicates ( ).

A: retention of damp-heat
B: invasion of damp-cold
C: invasion of summer heat
D: stagnation of both Qi and blood
E: deficiency of kidney yin

19. All the following syndromes may exhibit a pale tongue except ( ).

A: deficiency of blood
B: deficiency of Qi and blood
C: deficiency of yin
D: deficiency of yang
E: cold

20. A red tongue with a thick yellow coating indicates ( ).

A: excessive heat
B: deficient heat
C: retention of damp
D: stagnation of blood
E: stagnaiton of liver Qi

21. In exogenous febrile diseases, invasion of the ying and Xue (blood) systems by pathogenic heat may be indicated by ( ).

A: a pale tongue
B: a light red tongue
C: a deep red tongue
D: a purple tongue
E: a blue tongue

22. A pale tongue with a white slippery coating indicates ( ).

A: deficiency of Qi and blood
B: cold-damp
C: retention of food

D: invasion of summer heat
E: stagnation of Qi

23. A "geographic tongue" is a sign of ( ).
A: consumption of Qi and yin of the stomach
B: deficiency of Qi and heart blood
C: deficiency of yang of the spleen and kidney
D: deficiency of blood and yin of the liver
E: retention of phlegm-damp in the spleen and lung

24. A black and slippery coating implies ( ).
A: hyperactivity of fire due to deficiency of yin
B: excessive cold due to yang deficiency
C: retention of damp-heat
D: accumulation of fire
E: retention of food

25. A grey and dry coating implies ( ).
A: reteniton of cold-damp in the interior
B: retention of phlegm and fluid
C: consumption of body fluid due to excessive heat
D: excessive cold
E: yang deficiency

26. A thin, dry and deep red tongue indicates ( ).
A: hyperactivity of fire due to deficiency of yin
B: Qi deficiency
C: blood deficiency
D: deficiency of Qi and blood
E: excessive cold

27. Pale lips denote ( ).
A: retention of food
B: stagnation of blood
C: excessive heat
D: deficiency of blood
E: deficiency of yin

28. Clear nasal discharge is due to ( ).
A: invasion of wind-cold
B: invasion of wind-heat
C: deficiency of lung Qi

D: yin deficiency of the lung
E: retention of phlegm in the lung

29. Repeated speech in a feeble voice accompanied by listlessness suggests ( ).
A: disturbance of the mind by heat
B: deficiency of heart and lung Qi
C: disturbance of the mind by phlegm-fire
D: deficiency of heart blood
E: deficiency of spleen and lung Qi

30. Feeble asthmatic breathing accompanied by shortness of breath indicates ( ).
A: invasion of the lung by pathogenic wind-cold
B: invasion of the lung by pathogenic wind-heat
C: deficiency of lung Qi
D: deficiency of yin of the lung
E: retention of the phlegm in the lung

31. Alternate chills and fever are the representative symptoms of ( ).
A: exterior syndrome
B: interior syndrome
C: intermediate syndrome
D: heat syndrome
E: cold syndrome

32. Afternoon fever with constipation, as well as fullness and pain in the abdomen, often suggests ( ).
A: deficiency of yin
B: intermediate syndrome
C: invasion of pathogenic cold in the Taiyang channel
D: excess heat of the Yangming channel
E: stagnation of Qi and blood in the large intestine

33. Chills accompanied by fever is the symptom seen in ( ).
A: cold syndrome
B: heat syndrome
C: deficiency of yang
D: deficiency of yin
E: exterior syndrome

34. Severe chills accompanied by a mild fever suggests ( ).
A: deficiency of yang

B: deficiency of yin
C: exterior cold syndrome
D: exterior heat syndrome
E: interior cold syndrome

35. Absence of sweating in exteiror syndromes indicates ( ).
A: invasion by pathogenic wind
B: invasion by pathogenic cold
C: invasion by pathogenic heat
D: invasion by pathogenic damp
E: deficiency of yang

36. A sweet taste and stickiness in the mouth may imply ( ).
A: damp-heat in the spleen and stomach
B: heat in the liver and stomach
C: heat in the liver and gallbladder
D: cold in the spleen and stomach
E: liver qi overacting on the spleen

37. Sour regurgitation means ( ).
A: retention of heat in the liver and stomach
B: damp-heat in the spleen and stomach
C: yang deficiency of the spleen
D: cold in the liver channel
E: dysfunction of the spleen and stomach

38. A thin patient who is always hungry with a voracious appetite indicates ( ).
A: stagnation of spleen Qi
B: liver fire
C: excessive stomach fire
D: liver Qi overacting on the stomach
E: hyperactivity of yang due to deficiency of yin

39. Hunger with no appetite or eating a small amount of food suggests ( ).
A: weakness of the spleen due to deficiency of Qi
B: impairment of stomach yin producing internal heat of the deficiency type
C: excessive stomach fire
D: retention of undigestive food in the stomach
E: stagnation of stomach Qi due to overacting of the liver

40. A sharp, pricking pain which is in a fixed location is a sign of ( ).
A: yang deficiency

B: yin deficiency
C: stagnation of Qi
D: stagnation of blood
E: invasion of fire

41. Pain with a hollow sensation is caused by ( ).
A: deficiency of Qi
B: deficiency of yang
C: deficiency of blood
D: stagnation of Qi
E: retention of damp

42. A distending pain moving from place to place is a typical sign of ( ).
A: Qi stagnation
B: blood stagnation
C: cold syndrome
D: deficiency of blood
E: deficiency of Qi

43. Yellow urine generally indicates ( ).
A: cold syndromes
B: heat syndromes
C: deficiency of blood
D: deficiency of Qi
E: invasion of damp

44. Menses of a shortened cycle, excessive in amount, deep red in colour and thick in quality is related mainly to ( ).
A: weakness of spleen Qi which fails to control the blood
B: deficiency of blood
C: hyperactivity of fire due to deficiency of yin
D: excessive heat in blood
E: deficiency of the kidney which fails to store essence

45. A thin, light-coloured menstrual flow which is profuse indicates ( ).
A: excessive heat in blood
B: hyperactivity of fire due to deficiency of yin
C: failure of the spleen Qi to control blood
D: failure of the liver to store blood
E: dysfunction of the heart to dominate blood

46. Thin, scanty and light-coloured menstrual flow implies (   ).

A: deficiency of blood
B: deficiency of Qi
C: deficiency of yin
D: excessive heat in blood
E: stagnation of blood

47. A soft pulse (ru mai) is (   ).

A: superficial and thready, and hits the fingers without strength
B: deep and thready, and hits the fingers without strength
C: slow, with less than four beats per breath
D: felt only on heavy pressure
E: superficial and rapid

48. A broad, large and forceful pulse like roaring waves which come on powerfully and fade away is called (   ).

A: superficial pulse (*fu mai*)
B: deep pulse (*chen mai*)
C: pulse of the excess type (*chi mai*)
D: string-taut pulse (*xuan mai*)
E: surging pulse (*hong mai*)

49. A tight and forceful pulse like a stretched rope is called (   ).

A: surging pulse (*hong mai*)
B: slow pulse (*chi mai*)
C: rolling pulse (*hua mai*)
D: tense pulse (*jin mai*)
E: string-taut pulse (*xuan mai*)

50. A slow pulse with irregular missed beats is called (   ).

A: weak pulse (*ruo mai*)
B: soft pulse (*ru mai*)
C: hesitant pulse (*se mai*)
D: abrupt pulse (*cu mai*)
E: knotted pulse (*jie mai*)

51. The course of channel may present syndromes of the same organ when it is effected. The pathologic factors of the liver, for example, can be reflected by disorders at (   ).

A: the elbows
B: the fossae poplitea

C: the armpits (fossae axillaris)
D: the hips
E: none of the above

52. When the spleen is effected, disorders on each of the following areas would not be found except for ( ).

A: the elbows
B: the armpits
C: the hips
D: the fossae poplitea
E: none of the above

53. When a patient complains of ulceration, swelling and pain of the mouth and tongue, accompanied by insomnia, a feverish sensation, flushed face, bitter taste in the mouth, and hot and dark yellow urine, upon examination the patient exhibits a red tongue and rapid pulse, and the probable diagnosis would be ( ).

A: hyperactivity of the liver fire
B: deficiency of kidney yin
C: hyperactivity of heart fire
D: hyperactivity of urinary bladder fire
E: hyperactivity of stomach fire

54. Which one of the following symptoms could be an indication of points on the large intestine, small intestine, stomach and kidney channels in common? ( )

A: edema
B: toothache
C: sore throat
D: diarrhea
E: malar flush

V. Differentiation of Syndromes

1. An exterior syndrome can be differentiated by the presence of ( ).

A: tidal fever
B: high fever with aversion to heat
C: alternating chills and fever
D: chills and fever

E: chills without fever

2. An exterior deficiency syndrome can be differentiated by the presence of ( ).

A: chills
B: fever
C: sweating
D: thin tongue coating
E: superficial pulse

3. A patient has the following signs and symptoms: cough of one week in duration , severe chills with high fever, no sweating, red complexion, and yellow urine. The tongue has a thin coating and the pulse is superficial, rolling and rapid. This syndrome belongs to ( ).

A: exteiror heat syndrome
B: exterior cold syndrome
C: intermediate syndrome
D: exterior cold and interior heat syndrome
E: true cold with false heat syndrome

4. A patient has the following signs and symptoms: mild chills, fever, headache, cough, sore throat, loose stool and clear urine with an increased output. This syndrome belongs to ( ).

A: exterior heat and inteiror cold
B: true cold and false heat
C: exterior cold
D: exterior and interior deficiency
E: exteiror and interior cold

5. A patient has the following signs and symptoms: desire to cover up the body in spite of a feverish sensation, flushed face, thirst, drinking warm fluids, clear urinary output, and loose stools. The tongue is slightly purple with a moist white coating and the pulse is superficial and weak. This syndrome belongs to ( ).

A: true heat with false cold
B: true cold with false heat
C: exterior heat and inteiror cold
D: exterior cold and inteiror heat
E: hyperactivity of yang due to deficiency of yin

6. A cold syndrome frequently causes all of the following except ( ).

A: pallor
B: absence of thirst
C: preference for cold drinks
D: white and moist coating
E: increased urinary output which is clear

7. A heat syndrome frequently causes all of the following except ( ).

A: dark yellow and scanty urine
B: constipation
C: fever
D: dry tongue coating
E: absence of thirst

8. A patient has the following signs and symptoms: heat sensation in the chest, frequent desire to vomit, abdominal pain alleviated by warmth, and loose stools. This syndrome belongs to ( ).

A: cold above with heat below
B: heat above with cold below
C: true heat with false cold
D: true cold with false heat
E: exterior heat

9. A patient has the following signs and symptoms: cold extremities, thirst, preference for cold drinks, constipation, and scanty dark yellow urine. The tongue has a dry coating and the pulse is deep and forceful. This syndrome belongs to ( ).

A: exterior heat and interior cold
B: cold above with heat below
C: heat above with cold below
D: true cold with false heat
E: true heat with false cold

10. A patient has the following signs and symptoms: afternoon fever, malar flush , heat sensation of the palms and soles, night sweating, dryness of the throat and mouth, and dry stools. The tongue is red with little coating and the pulse is rapid. This syndrome belongs to ( ).

A: deficiency of yin
B: deficiency of yang
C: deficiency of Qi

D: deficiency of blood
E: deficiency of Qi and blood

11. A patient has the following signs and symptoms: chills, cold limbs, listlessness, lassitude, spontaneous sweating, increased urinary output which is clear, and loose stools. The tongue is pale and the pulse is weak. This syndrome belongs to ( ).

A: deficiency of Qi
B: deficiency of blood
C: deficiency of yang
D: deficiency of yin
E: deficiency of Qi and blood

12. An excess syndrome frequently causes all of the following except ( ).

A: resonant voice
B: distension and fullness in the chest and abdomen
C: pain aggravated by pressure
D: thick tongue coating
E: night sweating

13. A patient has the following signs and symptoms: aversion to speaking, lassitude, dizziness, spontaneous sweating. All symptoms become worse on exertion. The tongue is pale and the pulse is weak. This syndrome belongs to ( ).

A: deficiency of Qi
B: deficiency of blood
C: deficiency of yang
D: deficiency of yin
E: deficiency of Qi and blood

14. A patient has the following signs and symptoms: dizziness, lassitude, a bearing-down and distending sensation in the abdominal region, and prolapse of the anus. The tongue is pale and the pulse is weak. This syndrome belongs to ( ).

A: deficiency of Qi
B: deficiency of yang
C: stagnation of Qi
D: perversion of Qi
E: sinking of Qi

15. Stagnation of Qi can be differentiated by the presence of the following symptom ( ).

A: lassitude
B: hiccups
C: distending pain
D: hollow pain
E: bearing-down and distending sensation in the abodominal region

16. A patient has the following signs and symptoms: pale complexion, pale lips, dizziness, blurred vision, palpitation, insomnia, and numbness of the hands and feet. The tongue is pale and the pulse is thready. This syndrome belongs to ( ).

A: deficiency of Qi
B: deficiency of blood
C: deficiency of yang
D: deficiency of yin
E: sinking of Qi

17. Stagnation of blood frequently causes all of the following except ( ).

A: pain
B: tumour
C: hemorrhage
D: pale lips
E: ecchymosis

18. A young female patient has the following signs and symptoms: lower abdominal pain which usually starts before menstruation. The menstruation is delayed, scanty, and dark purple with clots. The tongue is purplish with purple spots on the edge and the pulse is deep. This syndrome belongs to ( ).

A: deficiency of blood
B: stagnation of Qi
C: stagnation of blood
D: deficiency of Qi
E: deficiency of yin

19. A patient has the following signs and symptoms: mental restlessness, bleeding, and a dry mouth with no desire to drink. The tongue is deep red and the pulse is rapid. This syndrome belongs to ( ).

A: stagnaiton of blood
B: heat in the blood

C: deficiency of blood
D: deficiency of yin
E: cold in the blood

20. A patient has the following signs and symptoms: dizziness, aversion to speaking, lassitude, and sharp pricking pain in the hypochondriac region. The tongue is pale with purple spots on the edge and the pulse is thready and string-taut. This syndrome belongs to ( ).

A: deficiency of Qi and blood
B: cold in the blood
C: deficiency of Qi and stagnation of blood
D: deficiency of yin and stagnation of blood
E: deficiency of yang and stagnation of blood

21. All of the following signs and symptoms may be due to deficiency of blood except ( ).

A: malar flush
B: blurring of vision and dizziness
C: palpitation and insomnia
D: numbness on the hands and feet
E: thready pulse

22. A patient has the following signs and symptoms: palpitation, shortness of breath becoming worse upon exertion, and fullness of the chest. The tongue is pale with a thin white coating and the pulse is thready and weak. This syndrome belongs to ( ).

A: deficiency of heart Qi
B: deficiency of heart yang
C: deficiency of heart blood
D: deficiency of lung Qi
E: invasion of the lung by pathogenic wind

23. A deficiency of heart yang and a deficiency of heart Qi can be differentiated by the presence of the following symptom ( ).

A: palpitation
B: shortness of breath
C: spontaneous sweating
D: chills
E: intermittent pulse

24. a patient has the following signs and symptoms: chills, cold limbs, palpitations, cardiac pain, and pale complexion. The tongue is pale, swollen with a white moist coating and the pulse is thready and weak. This syndrome belongs to ( ).

A: stagnation of heart blood
B: deficiency of heart Qi
C: deficiency of heart yang
D: deficiency of kidney yang
E: deficiency of heart blood

25. A patient has the following signs and symptoms: palpitation, insomnia, dream-disturbed sleep, poor memory, sensation of heat in palms of the hands and soles of the feet, and night sweating. The tongue is red and the pulse is thready and rapid. This syndrome belongs to ( ).

A: deficiency of heart blood
B: deficiency of heart yin
C: deficiency of liver blood
D: deficiency of liver yin
E: deficiency of lung yin

26. A patient has the following signs and symptoms: mental depression, dullness, incoherent speech, and weeping or laughing without an apparent reason. The tongue has a white sticky coating and the pulse is string taut and rolling. This syndrome belongs to ( ).

A: hyperactivity of heart fire
B: stagnation of heart blood
C: deficiency of heart blood
D: phlegm misting the heart
E: dificiency of heart yin

27. A patient has the following signs and symptoms: feeble cough, shortness of breath becoming worse upon exertion, clear dilute sputum, and spontaneous sweating. The tongue is pale with a thin white coating and the pulse is weak. This syndrome belongs to ( ).

A: invasion of the lung by pathogenic wind
B: deficiency of lung Qi
C: deficiency of the defensive Qi (Wei Qi)
D: retention of phlegm in the lung
E: deficiency of the primary Qi (Yuan Qi)

28. A patient has the following signs and symptoms: cough with white sticky sputum, fullness and stuffiness of the chest, and asthmatic breathing. The tongue has a white sticky coating and the pulse is rolling. This syndrome belongs to (   ).

A: invasion of the lung by pathogenic wind cold
B: invasion of the lung by pathogenic wind heat
C: retention of phlegm damp in the lung
D: retention of phlegm heat in the lung
E: deficiency of lung Qi

29. A patient has the following signs and symptoms: cough, chest pain with asthmatic breathing, and thick yellow sputum for one week. The tongue is red with a sticky yellow coating and the pulse is rolling and rapid. This syndrome belongs to (   ).

A: invasion of the lung by wind cold
B: stagnation of heart blood
C: retention of phlegm-damp in the heart
D: phlegm-fire disturbing the heart
E: retention of phlegm-heat in the lung

30. A patient has the following signs and symptoms: abdominal pain, diarrhea with blood and mucus in the stool for one day, scanty deep yellow urine and a burning sensation in the anus. The tongue has a sticky yellow coating and the pulse is rolling and rapid. This syndrome belongs to (   ).

A: invasion of the lung by pathogenic dryness
B: consumption of fluids in the large intestine
C: deficiency of lung yin
D: damp-heat in the large intestine
E: stagnation of Qi and the large intestine

31. Consumption of fluid in the large intestine frequently causes all the following except (   ).

A: dry stools
B: dryness in the mouth
C: constipation
D: dryness of the throat
E: voracious appetite

32. A patient has the following signs and symptoms: poor appetite, abdominal distension for three months, lassitude and aversion to speaking. The tongue

is pale with a thin white coating and the pulse is slow and weak. This syndrome belongs to (   ).

A: defiency of lung Qi
B: deficiency of heart Qi
C: deficiency of spleen Qi
D: deficiency of kidney Qi
E: deficiency of spleen and kidney yang

33. A patient has the following signs and symptoms: distention, fullness and pain of the epigastrium and abdomen, belching with a foul odour, and anorexia. The tongue has a thick and sticky coating and the pulse is rolling. This syndrome belongs to (   ).

A: damp-heat in the spleen and stomach
B: invasion of the spleen by cold-damp
C: deficiency of spleen Qi
D: retention of food in the stomach
E: deficiency of spleen and kidney yang

34. A patient has the following signs and symptoms: fullness and distension of the hypogastrium and abdomen, loss of appetite, sticky saliva, heaviness of the head and body, and loose stools. The tongue has a sticky white coating and the pulse is soft. This syndrome belongs to (   ).

A: deficiency of spleen Qi
B: deficiency of spleen yang
C: invasion of spleen by cold-damp
D: retention of food in the stomach
E: deficiency of stomach yin

35. Dysfunction of the spleen frequently causes all the following except (   ).

A: abdominal pain
B: foul belching and vomiting
C: loose stools
D: bleeding
E: edema

36. Deficiency of stomach yin can be differentiated by the presence of the following symptom (   ).

A: hunger with no desire to eat
B: vomiting and hiccups
C: dryness of the mouth and throat

D: constipation

E: pain in the epigastric region

37. A patient has the following signs and symptoms: burning sensation and pain in the epigastric region, sour regurgitation, empty and uncomfortable feeling in the stomach, easily hungry, thirst with a preference for cold drinks, and painful swelling of the gums. The tongue is red with a yellow coating and the pulse is rapid. This syndrome belongs to ( ).

A: hyperactivity of fire in the stomach

B: retention of food in the stomach

C: deficiency of stomach yin

D: damp-heat in the spleen and stomach

E: damp-heat in the large intestine

38. A female patient has the following signs and symptoms: pale complexion, lassitude, poor appetite, abdominal distension, excessive menstrual flow, and light red menses. The tongue is pale with a thin coating and the pulse is weak. This syndrome belongs to ( ).

A: heat in the blood

B: deficiency of spleen Qi

C: deficiency of spleen yang

D: dysfunction of the spleen in controlling blood

E: dysfunction of the liver in storing blood

39. A patient has the following signs and symptoms: hypochondriac distension and pain, bitter taste in the mouth, poor appetite, nausea, vomiting, and scanty yellow urine for one week. The tongue has a sticky yellow coating and the pulse is string-taut and rapid. This syndrome belongs to ( ).

A: damp-heat in the liver and gallbladder

B: damp-heat in the spleen and stomach

C: damp-heat in the bladder

D: damp-heat in the large intestine

E: stagnation of liver Qi

40. Deficiency of liver blood can be differentiated by the presence of the following symptom ( ).

A: pallor

B: nmumbness of the limbs and spasm of the tendons

C: dizziness and vertigo

D: palpitation and insomnia

E: pale tongue and thready pulse

41. Dysfunction of the liver frequently causes all of the following except ( ).

A: hypochondriac pain
B: irritability
C: dizziness and vertigo
D: spasm of the tendons
E: chills

42. A patient has the following signs and symptoms: mental depression, irritability, and distending pain in the costal and hypochodriac regions. This syndrome belongs to ( ).

A: stagnation of liver Qi
B: stagnation of liver blood
C: liver fire
D: damp-heat in the liver
E: retention of food

43. A patient has the following signs and symptoms: distending pain in the head, dizziness, vertigo, redness of the eyes, irritability, bitter taste and dryness of the mouth, yellow urine and constipation. The tongue is red with a yellow coating and the pulse is string taut and rapid. This syndrome belongs to ( ).

A: rising of liver yang
B: deficiency of liver yin
C: flare-up of liver fire
D: damp-heat in the liver
E: stagnation of liver Qi

44. A patient has the following signs and symptoms: headache with a distending sensation in the head, dizziness and vertigo, tinnitus, flushed face and red eyes, and irritability. Insomnia with dream-disturbed sleep, and soreness of the lower back. The tongue is red and the pulse is string-taut, thready and rapid. This syndrome belongs to ( ).

A: stagnation of liver fire
B: flare-up of liver fire
C: deficiency of liver blood
D: rising of liver yang
E: damp-heat in the liver

45. A patient has the following signs and symptoms: pallor, dizziness, tinnitus,

blurred vision, numbness of the hands and feet, and scanty light red menses. The tongue is pale and the pulse is weak and thready. This syndrome belongs to ( ).

A: deficiency of heart blood
B: deficiency of liver yin
C:deficiency of heart Qi
D: deficiency of kidney yin
E: none of the above

46. Dysfunction of the kidney frequently causes all of the following except ( ).

A: soreness and weakness of the lumbar region and knee joints
B: tinnitus and deafness
C: edema
D: impotence and infertility
E: fullness of the chest

47. A patient has the following signs and symptoms: soreness and weakness of the lumbar region and knee joints, frequent clear urination, and dribbling urine after urination. The tongue is pale with a white coating and the pulse is thready and weak. This syndrome belongs to ( ).

A: deficiency of kidney yin
B: deficiency of kidney Qi
C: damp-heat in the bladder
D: deficiency of liver yin
E: deficiency of spleen yang

48. Damp-heat in the bladder frequently causes all of the following except ( ).

A: frequency of urination
B: urgency of urination
C: burning pain in the urethra
D: yellow urine
E: enuresis

49. A patient has the following signs and symptoms: fever, lower abdominal distension, frequent and urgent urination, burning pain in the urethra, and yellow urine. The tongue has a sticky yellow coaitng and the pulse is rapid. This syndrome belongs to ( ).

A: hyperactivity of heart fire
B: damp-heat in the spleen and stomach
C: damp-heat in the liver

D: flare-up of liver fire
E: none of the above

50. A patient has the following signs and symptoms: distension and pain of the costal, hypochondriac and epigastric regions, belching, and acid regurgitation. This syndrome belongs to ( ).

A: stagnation of the liver
B: imbalance between the liver and spleen
C: disharmony between the liver and stomach
D: retention of food in the stomach
E: hyperactivity of stomach fire

51. Diarrhea at dawn is usually caused by ( ).

A: retention of fluid
B: imbalance between the liver and spleen
C: damp-heat in the large intestine
D: invasion of the spleen by cold-damp
E: yang deficiency of the spleen and kidney

52. Which of the following symptoms can be seen in either the cold syndrome of the excess type or the heat syndrome of the excess type? ( )

A: pallor
B: clear urine with increased volume
C: delirium
D: abdominal distention and pain aggravated by pressure
E: absence of thirst

53. Deficiency of yin frequently causes all of the following except ( ).

A: clear urine with increased volume
B: afternoon fever
C: insomnia with mental restlessness
D: night sweating
E: feverish sensation in palms and soles

54. A patient has the following signs and symptoms: palpitation, cardiac retardation and pain, and cyanosis of the lips and nails. This syndrome belongs to ( ).

A: deficiency of heart yin
B: deficiency of heart yang
C: deficiency of heart fire
D: stagnation of heart blood

E: stagnation of liver Qi

55. According to TCM pathology, the pathogen that is frequently seen in late autumn is ( ).

A: cold
B: wind
C: dryness
D: dampness
E: fire

56. Stagnant blood frequently causes all of the following except ( ).

A: pricking pain
B: hemorrhage
C: ecchymosis or petechia
D: mass tumour
E: soft and movable nodules

57. Each of the following signs may result from phlegm except ( ).

A: asthma
B: coma and rattle in the throat
C: hemiplegia
D: soft and movable nodules
E: pain

VI. Techniques of Acupuncture, Moxibustion and Cupping

1. Insertion of a needle by stretching the skin can be applied to ( ).

A: puncture with a long needle
B: puncture with a short needle
C: puncture those points where the skin is loose
D: puncture those points where the skin is thin
E: none of the above

2. Which of the following methods is suitable for puncturing with a short needle ? ( )

A: inserting the needle aided by the pressure of the finger of the pressing hand .

B: inserting the needle with the help of the puncturing and pressing hands.

C: inserting the needle with the fingers stretching the skin

D: inserting the needle by pinching the skin
E: none of the above

3. Zanzhu (B 2) and Yintang (Extra) should be punctured ( ).

A: with the fingers stretching the skin
B: with the fingers pinching the skin
C: with the help of the puncturing and pressing hands
D: using heavy pressure by fingers of the pressing hand
E: none of the above

4. All the following points should be punctured horizontally except ( ).

A: Touwei (S 8)
B: Zanzhu (B 2)
C: Zhongwan (Ren 12)
D: Yangbai (B 14)
E: Tanzhong (Ren 17)

5. All the following points should be punctured obliquely except ( ).

A: Lieque (L 7)
B: Jiuwei (Ren 15)
C: Shangxing (Du 23)
D: Touwei (S 8)
E: Feishu (B 13)

6. According to *Chinese Acupuncture and Moxibustion* the back "Shu" point located below the spinous process should be punctured ( ).

A: perpendicularly
B: obliquely
C: horizontally
D: subcutaneously
E: all of the above

7. Which of the following methods would you utilize to stimulate the points Jinjin (Extra) and Yuye (Extra)? ( )

A: puncturing perpendicularly
B: puncturing obliquely
C: puncturing horizontally
D: pricking to cause bleeding
E: moxibustion

8. Which of the following methods would you use to stimulate Shenque

(Ren 8)? ( )

A: puncturing perpendicularly
B: puncturing obliquely
C: puncturing horizontally
D: pricking to cause bleeding
E: moxibustion

9. According to *Chinese Acupuncture and Moxibustion* all the following are reinforcing methods except ( ).

A: lifting the needle gently and slowly
B: inserting the needle gently
C: keeping the hole closed
D: rotating the needle gently and slowly with small amplitude
E: rotating the needle forward with the thumb

10. All the following are reducing medhods except ( ).

A: pointing the tip of the needle against the channel course
B: lifting the needle forcefully and rapidly
C: setting the mountain on fire
D: thrusting the needle gently and slowly
E: keeping the hole open

11. The function of moxibustion is ( ).

A: to warm channels and expel cold
B: to induce the smooth flow of Qi and blood
C: to strengthen yang from collapse
D: to prevent diseases and maintain health
E: all of the above

12. Which of the following methods would you use first to treat a patient with excessive sweating, cold limbs and an undetectable pulse? ( )

A: moxibustion with ginger
B: moxibustion with garlic
C: moxibustion with salt
D: scarring moxibustion
E: none of the above

13. All the following points are often stimulated by pricking to cause bleeding except ( ).

A: ear apex
B: Weizhong (B 40)

C: Shixuan (Extra)
D: Hegu (LI 4)
E: Yintang (Extra)

14. Which of the following methods is appropriate for the point Ruzhong (S 17)? ( )

A: puncturing perpendicularly
B: puncturing subcutaneously
C: pricking to cause bleeding
D: moxibustion
E: none of the above

15. Which of the following methods is appropriate for the point Rugen (S 18)? ( )

A: puncturing obliquely 0.3-0.5 inch
B: puncturing perpendicularly 0.5-1 inch
C: priking to cause bleeding
D: all of the above
E: none of the above

16. According to *Chinese Acupuncture and Moxibustion* Jianjing (G 21) should be punctured ( ).

A: 0.3-0.5 inch perpendicularly
B: 0.5-0.8 inch horizontally
C: 0.8-1.5 inches perpendicularly
D: 0.8-0.9 inch obliquely
E: 0.9-1 inch obliquely

17. Needles should be sterilized in an autoclave at 1.5 atmospheric pressure and 125°C for ( ).

A: 10 minutes
B: 15 minutes
C: 20 minutes
D: 25 minutes
E: 30 minutes

18. All of the following diseases may be treated by cupping except ( ).

A: pain of the shoulders
B: pain of the lower back and leg
C: stomachache, vomiting and diarrhea
D: cough and asthma

E: spontaneous bleeding

19. According to *Chinese Acupuncture and Moxibustion* the point Yamen (Du 15) should be punctured ( ).

A: 0.3-0.5 inch upward obliquely
B: 0.5-0.8 inch perpendicularly
C: 0.5-0.8 inch upward obliquely
D: 0.8-1 inch perpendicularly
E: 0.8-1 inch upward obliquely

20. Grain-like intradermal needle should not be imbedded into the point ( ).

A: Xinshu (UB 15)
B: Shenmen (H 7)
C: Ruzhong (S 17)
D: Zusanli (St 36)
E: Dazhui (Du 14)

21. In treating disorders on the trunk, from which area of the auricle should points be selected? ( )

A: cymba conchae
B: helix crus
C: antihelix
D: lobule
E: cavum conchae

22. An inappropriate auricular point for treating diarrhea is ( ).

A: the large intestine point
B: the small intestine point
C: the sympathetic point
D: the spleen point
E: the heart point

23. In which of the following circumstances should you not utilize a three-edged needle? ( )

A: sudden loss of consciousness caused by high-grade fever
B: apoplexy
C: sunstroke
D: swelling and pain of eyes
E: palpitation and insomnia

VII. Treatment of Diseases

1. The Xi-Cleft point of the stomach channel is (   ).

A: Fenglong (S 40)
B: jiexi (S 41)
C: Liangqiu (S 34)
D: Chongyang (S 42)
E: Xiangu (S 43)

2. Each of the following points is the Xi-Cleft point except (   ).

A: Gongsun (SP 4)
B: Kongzui (L 6)
C: Ximen (P 4)
D: Zhongdu (Liv 6)
E: Shuiquan (K 5)

3. All the following points are one of the eight confluent points except (   ).

A: Zhaohai (K 6)
B: Yuji (L 10)
C: Zulinqi (G 41)
D: Waiguan (SJ 5)
E: Shenmai (B 62)

4. Which of the following points is the Xi-Cleft point for the Yangqiao channel? (   )

A: Jiaoxin (K 8)
B: Gongsun (Sp 4)
C: Shuiquan (K 5)
D: Fuyang (B 59)
E: Zhubin (K 9)

5. Which of the following points is the Xi-Cleft points for the Yinwei channel? (   )

A: Liangqiu (S 34)
B: Waiqiu (G 36)
C: Jinmen (B 63)
D: Shuiquan (K 5)
E: none of the above

6. The influential point for Qi is (   ).

A: Qihu (S 13)

B: Qihai (Ren 6)
C: Qishi (S 11)
D: Qixue (K 13)
E: none of the above

7. Which of the following points is not a Xi-Cleft point? (   )
A: Fuyang (B 59)
B: Jiaoxin (K 8)
C: Yangjiao (G 35)
D: Yangfu (G 38)
E: Zhubin (K 9)

8. Shenmai (B 62) is the eighth confluent point of (   ).
A: the Du channel
B: the Dai channel
C: the Yangqiao channel
D: the Yangwei channel
E: the Chong channel

9. The lower He-Sea point of the small intestine is (   ).
A: Shangjuxu (S 37)
B: Xiajuxu (S 39)
C: Zusanli (S 36)
D: Weizhong (B 40)
E: Weiyang (B 39)

10. All the following points are lower He-Sea points except (   ).
A: Shangjuxu (S 37)
B: Yanglingquan (G 34)
C: Weizhong (B 40)
D: Weiyang (B 39)
E: Qiuxu (G 40)

11. According to the principle of reinforcing the "mother" point for the deficient syndromes, which of the following points is the best selection for treating a deficient syndrome of the kidney? (   )
A: Yongquan (K 1)
B: Rangu (K 2)
C: Taixi (K 3)
D: Fuliu (K 7)
E: Yingu (K 10)

12. According to the principle of reinforcing the "mother" point for a deficient syndrome, which of the following points is the best selection for treating a deficient syndrome of the liver? ( )

A: Sanyinjiao (SP 6)
B: Taixi (K 3)
C: Yingu (K 10)
D: Dadu (Sp 2)
E: Taichong (Liv 3)

13. According to the principle of reducing the "son" point for an excess syndrome, which of the following points is the best selection for treating an excess syndrome of the gallbladder? ( )

A: Zuqiaoyin (G 44)
B: Xiaxi (G 43)
C: Zulinqi (G 41)
D: Yangfu (G 38)
E: Yanglingquan (G 34)

14. According to the principle of reducing the "son" point for an excess syndrome, which of the following points is the best selection for treating an excess syndrome of the heart? ( )

A: Shaochong (H 9)
B: Shaofu (H 8)
C: Shenmen (H 7)
D: Lingdao (H 4)
E: Shaohai (H 3)

15. According to the theory of the Five Elements, all the following points belong to metal except ( ).

A: Yangxi (LI 5)
B: Guanchong (SJ 1)
C; Lidui (S 45)
D: Jingqu (L 8)
E: Zhongfeng (Liv 4)

16. All the following points are the Luo-Connecting points except ( ).

A: Pianli (LI 6)
B: Lougu (SP 7)
C; Fenglong (S 40)
D: Feiyang (B 58)

E: Guangming (G 37)

17. All the following points are Front-Mu points except ( ).

A: Zhongji (Ren 3)
B: Jingmen (G 25)
C: Qihai (Ren 6)
D: Riyue (G 24)
E: Shimen (Ren 5)

18. Which of the following points is the Front-Mu point for the pericardium? ( )

A: Zhongfu (L 1)
B: Tanzhong (Ren 17)
C: Juque (Ren 14)
D: Shimen (Ren 5)
E: Qimen (Ren 14)

19. The influential point of Zang organs is ( ).

A: Zhongwan (Ren 12)
B: Zhangmen (Liv 13)
C: Tanzhong (Ren 17)
D: Dazhu (B 11)
E: none of the above

20. Which of the following prescriptions is the best for treating abdominal pain caused by the retention of food? ( )

A: Zhongwan (Ren 12), Shenque (Ren 8), Zusanli (S 36), Gongsun (Sp 4)
B: Zhongwan (Ren 12), Pishu (B 20), Weishu (B 21), Zusanli (S 36)
C: Zhongwan (Ren 12), Qihai (Ren 6), Zhangmen (Liv 13), Zusanli (S 36)
D: Zhongwan (Ren 12), Qihai (Ren 6), Guanyuan (Ren 4), Shenque (Ren 8)
E: Zhongwan (Ren 12), Tianshu (S 25), Zusanli (S 36), Inner-Neiting (Extra)

21. Which of the following prescriptions is the best for treating abdominal pain caused by the accumulation of cold? ( )

A: Zhongwan (Ren 12), Qimen (Liv 14), Yanglingquan (G 34), Zusanli (S 36)
B: Zhongwan (Ren 12), Qihai (Ren 6), Zhangmen (Liv 13), Zusanli (S 36)
C: Zhongwan (Ren 12), Shenque (Ren 8), Zusanli (S 36), Gongsun (Sp 4)
D: Zhongwan (Ren 12), Pishu (B 20), Weishu (B 21), Zusanli (S 36)
E: Zhongwan (Ren 12), Tianshu (S 25), Inner-Neiting (Extra), Zusanli (S 36)

22. The best prescription for a patient who complains of dizziness, irritability, flushed face, red eyes, tinnitus, bitter taste in the mouth and dream-disturbed sleep would be ( ).

A: Baihui (DU 20), Pishu (B 20), Guanyuan (Ren 4), Sanyinjiao (Sp 6)
B: Touwei (S 8), Pishu (B 20), Zhongwan (Ren 12), Neiguan (P 6)
C: Fenglong (S 40), Pishu (B 20), Neiguan (P 6), Sanyinjiao (Sp 6)
D: Guanyuan (Ren 4), Qihai (Ren 6), Shenshu (B 23), Zusanli (S 36)
E: Fengchi (G 20), Xingjian (Liv 2), Taixi (K 3), Ganshu (B 18)

23. Which of the following prescriptions is the best for treating a patient who complains of dizziness with a heavy feeling in the head and a suffocating sensation in the chest, nausea, profuse sputum, anorexia and sommol-ence? ( )

A: Fenglong (S 40), Neiguan (P 6), Pishu (B 20), Touwei (S 8)
B: Fengchi (G 20), Xingjian (Liv 2), Taichong (Liv 3), Ganshu (B 18)
C: Fengchi (G 20), Taixi (K 3), Shenshu (B 23), Ganshu (B 18)
D: Touwei (S 8), Pishu (B 20), Sanyinjiao (Sp 6), Zusanli (S 36)
E: Guanyuan (Ren 4), Qihai (Ren 6), Shenshu (B 23), Pishu (B 20)

24. Which of the following prescriptions is the best for treating a patient suffering from a common cold of the wind-heat type? ( )

A: Fengfu (Du 16), Fengmen (B 12), Fengchi (G 20), Lieque (L 7)
B: Hegu (LI 4), Lieque (L 7), Fenglong (S 40), Neiguan (P 6)
C: Taiyuan (L 9), Zhongfu (L 1), Feishu (B 13), Lieque (L 7)
D: Dazhui (Du 14), Quchi (LI 11), Hegu (LI 4), Yuji (L 10), Shaoshang (L 11)
E: Fengfu (Du 16), Fengmen (B 12), Fengchi (G 20), Feishu (B 13)

25. Which of the following is the best prescription for treating a patient who complains of chills, fever, headache, soreness and pain in the limbs, nasal obstruction, running nose, cough, no sweaitng, profuse thin sputum, a thin, white tongue coating, and a superficial and tense pulse? ( )

A: Dazhui (Du 14), Quchi (LI 11), Hegu (LI 4), Shaoshang (L 11)
B: Dazhui (Du 14), Quchi (LI 11), Hegu (LI 4), Waiguan (SJ 5)
C: Lieque (L 7), Fengchi (G 20), Fengmen (B 12), Hegu (LI 4)
D: Fengchi (G 20), Waiguan (SJ 5), Fenglong (S 40), Yingxiang (LI 20)
E: Feishu (B 13), Taiyang (Extra), Taodao (Du 13), Fenglong (S 40)

26. Which of the following points is the best selection for treating asthma of the wind-cold type? ( )

A: Fengmen (B 12)

B: Shenshu (K 23)
C: Qihai (Ren 6)
D: Shanzhong (Ren 17)
E: Taixi (K 3)

27. Which of the following points is the best selection for treating diarrhea caused by the deficiency of kidney yang? ( )

A: Sanyinjiao (Sp 6)
B: Tianshu (S 25)
C: Mingmen (Du 4)
D: Zusanli (St 36)
E: Yinlingquan (Sp 9)

28. A middle-aged patient has the following signs and symptoms: headache, painful joints, nasal obstruction, rhinorrhea, itching of the throat, cough, a thin expectoration, aversion to cold, a thin, white tongue coating, and a superficial and tense pulse. The best prescription at this time is ( ).

A: Dazhui (Du 14), Quchi (LI 11), Hegu (LI 4), Shixuan (Extra)
B: Dazhui (Du 14), Quchi (LI 11), Hegu (LI 4), Feishu (B 13)
C: Lieque (L 7), Fengchi (G 20), Fengmen (B 12), Waiguan (SJ 5)
D: Yingxiang (LI 20), Fengchi (G 20), Waiguan (SJ 5), Fenglong (St 40)
E: Taiyang (L 9), Feishu (B 13), Taodao (Du 13), Fenglong (St 40)

29. A patient has the following signs and ysmptoms: fever, headache, yellow phlegm, dry mouth, sore throat, a thin, yellow tongue coating, and a superficial and rapid pulse. The best prescription for him is ( ).

A: Feishu (B 13), Lieque (L 7), Dazhui (Du 14), Hegu (LI 4), Waiguan (SJ 5)
B: Chize (L 5), Shaoshang (L 11), Hegu (LI 4), Yuji (L 10), Waiguan (SJ 5)
C: Feishu (B 13), Taiyuan (L 9), Zhangmen (Liv 13), Taibai (Sp 2)
D: Feishu (B 13), Fenglong (St 40), Taiyuan (L 9), Taibai (Sp 2)
E: Feishu (B 13), Zhongfu (L 1), Lieque (L 7), Tanzhong (Ren 17)

30. In treating a cough caused by damp-phlegm, which of the following points should be punctured in addition to Feishu (B 13)? ( ).

A: Lieque (L 7) and Hegu (LI 4)
B: Dazhui (Du 14) and Shaoshang (L 11)
C: Fenglong (St 40) and Chize (L 5)
D: Chize (L 5) and Taichong (Liv 3)
E: Zhongfu (L 1) and Zhaohai (K 6)

31. In treating a cough caused by the lung being attacked by liver fire, which

-- the following prescriptions is the best selection? (   )

A: Ganshu (B 18), Yuji (L 10), Xingjian (Liv 2), Fengchi (G 20)
B: Feishu (B 13), Chize (L 5), Taichong (Liv 3), Xingjian (Liv 2)
C: Zhongfu (L 1) Feishu (B 13), Taiyuan (L 9), Zhaohai (K 6)
D: Lieque (L 7), Hegu (LI 4), Qimen (Liv 14), Ganshu (B 18)
E: Ganshu (B 18), Feishu (B 13), Fenglong (St 40), Zusanli (St 36)

32. The prescription composed of Zhongwan (Ren 12), Zusanli (St 36), Neiguan (P 6), Gongsun (Sp 4) and Taichong (Liv 3) is commonly used to treat vomiting caused by (   ).

A: pathogenic heat in the stomach
B: obstruction of food
C: pathogenic dampness in the stomach
D: deficiency of the spleen and stoamch
E: the stomach being attacked by liver Qi

33. The best prescription utilized to stop hiccups is (   ).

A: Tiantu (Ren 22), Tanzhong (Ren 17), Hegu (LI 4), Zusanli (St 36)
B: Tanzhong (Ren 17), Zhongwan (Ren 12), Weishu (B 21), Neiguan (P 6)
C: Geshu (B 17), Zhongwan (Ren 12), Neiguan (P 6), Zusanli (St 36)
D: Zhongwan (Ren 12), Neiguan (P 6), Ganshu (B 18), Zusanli (St 36)
E: Qihai (Ren 6), Zhongwan (Ren 12), Taichong (Liv 3), Tanzhong (Ren 17)

34. A patient has the following signs and symptoms: dribbling urination, attenuation in the force of the urine discharge, listlessness, a cold feeling below the waist, and weakness of the loins and knees. Examination shows a pale tongue and a deep, thready pulse weak at the Chiregion. The prescription of choice at this stage is (   ).

A: Pangguangshu (B 28), Yinlingquan (Sp 9), Zhongji (Ren 3), Weiyang (B 39)
B: Sanyinjiao (Sp 6), Yinlingquan (Sp 9), Zhongji (Ren 3), Zusanli (S 36)
C: Mingmen (Du 4), Shenshu (B 23), Guanyuan (Ren 4), Baihui (Du 20)
D: Zhongji (Ren 3), Dahe (K 12), Qugu (Ren 2), Shuiquan (K 5)
E: Shuidao (S 28), Pangguangshu (B 28), Weiyang (B 39), Shuifen (Ren 9)

35. Acupuncture at the points Zhongwan (Ren 12), Zusanli (S 36), Neiguan (P 6), Shenmen (H 7) and Sanyinjiao (Sp 6) is often used to treat insomnia caused by (   ).

A: deficiency of the heart and spleen
B: flare-up of fire resulting from a deficiency of yin

C: dysfunction of the stomach
D: disharmony between the heart and kidney
E: hyperactivity of liver yang

36. The best prescription for dizziness caused by hyperactivity of liver yang is ( ).

A: Pishu (B 20), Shenshu (B 23), Guanyuan (Ren 4) and Zusanli (S 36)
B: Baihui (Du 20), Qihai (Ren 6), Xuehai (SP 10) and Neiguan (P 6)
C: Ganshu (B 18), Shenshu (B 23), Xingjian (Liv 2) and Fengchi (G 20)
D: Sanyinjiao (Sp 6), Zusanli (S 36), Neiguan (P 6) and Fenglong (S 40)
E: Shenmen (H 7), Baihui (Du 20), Neiguan (P 6) and Zhongwan (Ren 12)

37. The best prescription for treatment of dizziness caused by the internal retention of phlegm-damp is ( ).

A: Pishu (B 20) Shenshu (B 23), Guanyuan (Ren 4), Zusanli (St 36)
B: Dazhui (Du 14), Baihui (Du 20), Sanyinjiao (Sp 6), Zusanli (St 36)
C: Pishu (B 20), Fenglong (S 40), Touwei (S 8), Zhongwan (Ren 12)
D: Fengchi (G 20), Feishu (B 13), Lieque (L 7), Baihui (Du 20)
E: Shenshu (B 23), Ganshu (B 18), Xingjian (Liv 2), Fengchi (G 20)

38. Which of the following prescriptions is the best selection for treating jaundice of the yin type? ( )

A: Yinlingquan (Sp 9), Pishu (B 20), Ganshu (B 18), Zusanli (St 36), Danshu (B 19)
B: Pishu (B 20), Ganshu (B 18), Danshu (B 19), Shenshu (B 23), Weishu (B 21)
C: Yinlingquan (Sp 9), Zusanli (S 36), Ganshu (B 18), Danshu (B 19), Yanglingquan (G 34)
D: Yinlingquan (Sp 9), Yanglingquan (G 34), Taichong (Liv 3), Pishu (B 20)
E: Yanglingquan (G 34), Taichong (Liv 3), Xingjian (Liv 2), Neiguan (P 6), Neiting (S 44)

39. Apart from the main points such as Yinlingquan (Sp 9), Ganshu (B 18), Danshu (B 19), Zhiyang (Du 9) and Zusanli (S 36), which of the following points would you use to treat jaundice of the yang type? ( )

A: Pishu (B 20) and Yanggang (B 48)
B: Yanglingquan (G 34) and Taichong (Liv 3)
C: Xingjian (Liv 2) and Taichong (Liv 3)
D: Hegu (LI 4) and Quchi (LI 11)
E: Neiting (S 44) and Quchi (LI 11)

40. The best prescription for treatment of jaundice of the yang type is ( ).

A: Shenshu (B 23), Pishu (B 20), Zhongwan (Ren 12), Zusanli (S 36), Zhiyang (Du 9)

B: Danshu (B 19), Yanglingquan (G 34), Yinlingquan (Sp 9), Neiting (S 44), Taicho ng (Liv 3), Ganshu (B 18)

C: Zhongwan (Ren 12), Zusanli (St 36), Neiguan (P 6), Tianshu (S 25), Sanyinjiao (Sp 6)

D: Mingmen (Du 4), Qihai (Ren 6), Shenshu (B 23), Sanyinjiao (Sp 6), Zusanli (S 36)

E: Ganshu (B 18), Pishu (B 20), Yinlingquan (Sp 9), Zhongwan (Ren 12), Danshu (B 19)

41. In addition to the main points such as Yinlingquan (Sp 9), Zusanli (S 36), Ganshu (B 18), and Danshu (B 19), which of the following points would you select in the treatment of jaundice? ( )

A: Mingmen (Du 4)

B: Qihai (Ren 6)

C: Dazhui (Du 14)

D: Pishu (B 20)

E: Zhiyang (Du 9)

42. Apart from the main points such as Dachangshu (B 25), Tianshu (S 25) and Zhigou (SJ 6), which of the following points would you use to treat constipation? ( )

A: Zhaohai (K 6)

B: Pishu (B 20)

C: Weishu (B 21)

D: Taixi (K 3)

E: Zhongwan (Ren 12)

43. Which of the following prescriptions is the best choice to treat a patient with the following signs and symptoms: infrequent and difficult defecation every three to five days (sometime longer), fullness and distending pain in the abdomen and hypochondriac regions, frequent belching, loss of appetite, a thin, sticky tongue coating and a string-taut pulse? ( )

A: Dachangshu (B 25), Tianshu (S 25), Zhaohai (K 6), Zhongwan (Ren 12), Zusanli (S 36)

B: Dachangshu (B 25), Tianshu (S 25), Zhigou (SJ 6), Zhongwan (Ren 12), Taichong (Liv 3)

C: Dachangshu (B 25), Tianshu (S 25), Quchi (LI 11), Hegu (LI 4), Zusanli (S 36)

D: Dachangshu (B 25), Tianshu (S 25), Pishu (B 20), Weishu (B 21), Zusanli (S 36)

E: Dachangshu (B 25), Tianshu (S 25), Qihai (Ren 6), Shenque (Ren 8), Zhongwan (Ren 12)

44. Apart from the main points such as Dachangshu (B 25) and Tianshu (S 25) employed in dealing with constipation caused by an accumulation of cold, which of th e following points would you use as secondary points? (   )

A: Zusanli (S 36) and Sanyinjiao (SP 6)

B: Quchi (LI 11) and Hegu (LI 4)

C: Shenque (Ren 8) and Qihai (Ren 6)

D: Taichong (Liv 3) and Zhigou (SJ 6)

E: Zhaohai (K 6) and Taixi (K 3)

45. An elderly patient has the following signs and symptoms: constipation, lassi tude, shortness of breath, dizziness, palpitation, pale and lustreless complexion, lips and nails, a pale tongue with a thin coating, and a thready and weak pulse. Which of the following methods would you use to treat this case? (   )

A: eliminating heat

B: moistening the intestines

C: removing the Qi stagnation

D: reinforcing the Qi and blood

E: warming the yang to dispel the cold

46. The best prescription for treatment of lower back pain is (   ).

A: Shenshu (B 23), Yaoyangguan (Du 3) and Weizhong (B 40)

B: Taixi (K 3), Fuliu (K 7) and Shenshu (B 23)

C: Mingmen (Du 4), Guanyuan (Ren 4) and Guanyuanshu (B 26)

D: Dachangshu (B 25), Guanyuanshu (B 26) and Zhishi (B 52)

E: Renzhong (Du 26), Yaotongxue (Extra) and Yaoyan (Extra)

47. In addition to the main points such as Shenshu (B 23), Yaoyangguan (Du 3) and Weizhong (B 40), which of the following points would you use to treat lower back pain due to traumatic injury? (   )

A: Taixi (K 3)

B: Mingmen (Du 4)

C: Renmzhong (Du 26)

D: Fuliu (K 7)
E: Zhishi (B 52)

48. Which of the following points would you utillize as secondary points to treat lower back pain caused by a deficiency of the kidney yang? ( )

A: Dachangshu (B 25) and Guanyuanshu (B 26)
B: Mingmen (Du 4) and Yaoyan (Extra)
C: Zhishi (B 52) and Taixi (K 3)
D: Renzhong (Du 26) and Yaotongxue (Extra)
E: Guanyuan (Ren 4) and Fuliu (K 7)

49. Choose the best prescription fora patient with the following signs and symptoms: insomnia, dream-disturbed sleep, dizziness, palpitation, poor memory, spontaneous sweating, anorexia, lassitude, a pale tongue with a thin coating, and a thready, weak pulse ( ).

A: Taixi (K 3), Shenmen (H 7), Shenshu (B 23), Sanyinjiao (Sp 6)
B: Sanyinjiao (Sp 6), Shenshu (B 23), Zusanli (S 36), Neiguan (P 6)
C: Sanyinjiao (Sp 6), Dadun (Liv 1), Guanyuan (Ren 4), Baihui (Du 20)
D: Sanyinjiao (Sp 6), Shenmen (H 7), Pishu (B 20), Xinshu (B 15)
E: Sanyinjiao (Sp 6), Shenmen (H 7), Fenglong (S 40), Weishu (B 21)

50. The best points for the treatment of insomnia are ( ).

A: Pishu (B 20), Xinshu (B 15) and Yinbai (Sp 1)
B: Xinshu (B 15), Shenshu (B 23) and Taixi (K 3)
C: Ganshu (B 18), Danshu (B 19) and Wangu (G 12)
D: Weishu (B 21), Fenglong (S 40) and Zusanli (S 36)
E: Shenmen (H 7), Sanyinjiao (Sp 6) and Anmian (Extra)

51. The most commonly used points for the treatment of palpitation are ( ).

A: Xinshu (B 15), Shenmen (H 7), Neiguan (P 6) and Juque (Ren 14)
B: Tongli (P 5), Qiuxu (G 40), Fenglong (S 40), and Danshu (B 19)
C: Pishu (B 20), Weishu (B 21) and Zusanli (S 36)
D: Jueyinshu (B 14), Shenshu (B 23) and Taixi (K 3)
E: Shuifen (Ren 9), Guanyuan (Ren 4), Shenque (Ren 8) and Yinlingquan (SP 9)

52. Apart from the main points such as Shenmen (H 7), Xinshu (B 15) and Neiguan (P 6), which of the following points would you select as supplementary points to treat palpitation due to the retention of pathogenic fluid? ( )

A: Tongli (P 5) and Qiuxu (G 40)
B: Shuifen (Ren 9), Guanyuan (Ren 4) and Yinlingquan (Sp 9)

C: Zusanli (S 36) and Sanyinjiao (Sp 6)
D: Fenglong (S 40) and Tiantu (Ren 22)
E: Taixi (K 3) and Fuliu (K 7)

53. Which of the following points would you select as the supplementary points to treat a patient with the following signs and symptoms: palpitations, tinnitus, dizziness, blurred vision, very little tongue coating, and a thready, rapid pulse? (   )

A: Fenglong (S 40) and Neiting (S 44)
B: Danshu (B 19) and Yanglingquan (G 34)
C: Shuifen (Ren 9) and Yinlingquan (Sp 9)
D: Taixi (K 3) and Shenshu (B 23)
E: Zusanli (S 36) and Pishu (B 20)

54. The prescription formed by Zhongji (Ren 3), Guilai (S 29), Xuehai (Sp 10), Taichong (Liv 3), Hegu (LI 4) and Sanyinjiao (Sp 6) is most appropriate to treat (   ).

A: dysmenorrhea of the excess type
B: dysmenorrhea of the deficient type
C: irregular menstruation
D: amenorrhea caused by blood depletion
E: amenorrhea caused by blood stagnation

55. Which of the following prescriptions is most commonly used to treat a cough due to the invasion by exogenous pathogens? (   )

A: Feishu (B 13), Zhongfu (L 1), Lieque (L 7) and Zhaohai (K 6)
B: Lieque (L 7), Hegu (LI 4) and Feishu (B 13)
C: Dazhui (Du 14), Waiguan (SJ 5) and Fengchi (G 20)
D: Hegu (LI 4), Chize (L 5) and Yuji (L 10)
E: Feishu (B 13), Chize (L 5), Zusanli (S 36) and Fenglong (S 40)

56. Apart from Feishu (B 13), Zhongfu (L 1) and Lieque (L 7), which of the following points would you consider the main point to treat a cough due to the deficiency of lung yin? (   )

A: Chize (L 5)
B: Taiyuan (L 9)
C: Yuji (L 10)
D: Zhaohai (K 6)
E: Taixi (K 3)

57. Shaoshang (L 11) can be selected as a supplementary point to treat a

cough accompanied by ( ).

A: fever

B: aversion to cold

C: pain and swelling of the throat

D: headache

E: dryness of the nose

58. Which of the following points would you select to treat a patient with a cough who is spitting blood or even coughing blood? ( )

A: Dazhui (Du 14) and Waiguan (SJ 5)

B: Kongzui (L 6) and Geshu (B 17)

C: Shaoshang (L 11) and Shangyang (LI 1)

D: Hegu (LI 4) and Quchi (LI 11)

E: Sanyinjiao (Sp 6) and Zhongfu (L 1)

59. Which of the following points are used to treat a cough by utilizing cupping ? ( )

A: Fengmen (B 12) and Feishu (B 13)

B: Chize (L 5) and Quchi (LI 11)

C: Dazhui (Du 14) and Taodao (Du 13)

D: Hegu (LI 4) and Shaoshang (LU 11)

E: Zusanli (S 36) and Sanyinjiao (Sp 6)

60. Which of the following channels would you use first to treat cough by tapping method with a cutaneous needle? ( )

A: Ren and Du channels

B: Lung and spleen channels

C: Du and bladder channels

D: kidney and Ren channels

E: none of the above

61. The prescription of Feishu (B 13), Chize (L 5) and Fenglong (S 40) can be used to treat cough caused by ( ).

A: invasion of cold

B: invasion of heat

C: dryness of the lung with a deficiency of yin

D: blockage of the lung by phlegm

E: weakness of the lung and kidney

62. Which of the following points is the principal point for the treatment of

asthma? (   )

A: Tiantu (Ren 22)
B: Fenglong (S 40)
C: Feishu (B 13)
D: Taibai (S 3)
E: Taiyuan (L 9)

63. A patient has the following signs and symptoms: short and rapid breathing, strong and coarse voice, cough with thick yellow sputum, fever, restlessness, stuffiness of the chest, a thick yellow coating on the tongue, and a rolling and rapid pulse. The best prescription of points at this stage in the disease is (   ).

A: Feishu (B 13), Fengmen (B 12), Dazhui (Du 14) and Hegu (LI 4)
B: Feishu (B 13), Dingchuan (Extra), Chize (L 5) and Fenglong (S 40)
C: Feishu (B 13), Taiyuan (L 9), Zusanli (S 36) and Taibai (Sp 3)
D: Taixi (K 3), Shenshu (B 23), Feishu (B 13) and Tanzhong (Ren 17)
E: Shenshu (B 23), Feishu (B 13), Pishu (B 20) and Taiyuan (L 9)

64. Using moxibustion, which of the following points have proved effective in the treatment of persistent asthma? (   )

A: Taiyuan (L 9) and Lieque (L 7)
B: Taixi (K 3) and Shenshu (B 23)
C: Tanzhong (Ren 17) and Qihai (Ren 6)
D: Shenzhu (Du 12) and Gaohuangshu (B 43)
E: Pishu (B 20) and Zhongwan (Ren 12)

65. Each of the following points may be selected to treat asthma due to the deficiency of the kidney except (   ).

A: Feishu (B 13)
B: Shenshu (B 23)
C: Taixi (K 3)
D: Qihai (Ren 6)
E: Chize (L 5)

66. All the following points can treat asthma due to wind-cold except (   ).

A: Feishu (B 13)
B: Fengmen (B 12)
C: Dazhui (Du 14)
D: Taiyuan (L 9)
E: Hegu (LI 4)

67. A young patient has the following signs and symtoms: distending pain in the epigastrium which is aggravated on pressure or after meals, belching with fetid odour, annorexia, a thick, sticky tongue coating, and a deep forceful pulse. The best prescription at this time is ( ).

A: Qimen (Liv 14), Zhongwan (Ren 12), Neiguan (P 6), Zusanli (S 36)
B: Jianli (Ren 11), Neiguan (P 6), Zusanli (S 36), Inner-Neiting (Extra)
C: Zhongwan (Ren 12), Qihai (Ren 6), Pishu (B 20), Zusanli (S 36)
D: Neiguan (P 6), Gongsun (Sp 4), Zhongwan (Ren 12), Pishu (B 20)
E: Taichong (Liv 3), Neiting (S 44), Hegu (LI 4), Zusanli (S 36)

68. The prescription of Qimen (Liv 14), Zhongwan (Ren 12), Neiguan (P 6), Zusanli (S 36) and Taichong (Liv 3) is used to treat epigastric pain caused by ( ).

A: Retention of food
B: deficiency of the stomach and spleen
C: accumulation of cold
D: attack of the stomach by liver Qi
E: deficiency of spleen yang

69. All the following points are principal points for the treatment of vomiting except ( ).

A: Zhongwan (Ren 12)
B: Zusanli (Ren 36)
C: Neiguan (P 6)
D: Taichong (Liv 3)
E: Gongsun (Sp 4)

70. Taichong (Liv 3) can be selected as a supplementary point to treat vomiting due to ( ).

A: retention of food
B: deficiency of spleen and stomach Qi
C: attack of the stomach by liver Qi
D: accumulation of cold at the stoamch
E: invasion of the stomach by heat

71. Which of the following prescriptions do you consider as the best one for a patient complaining of vomiting, loss of appetite, lassitude, weakness, and slightly loose stool? ( )

A: Zhongwan (Ren 12), Gongsun (Sp 4), Neiguan (P 6), Pishu (B 20), Weishu (B 21)

B: Zhongwan (Ren 12), Gongsun (Sp 4), Neiguan (P 6), Taichong (Liv 3)
C: Zhongwan (Ren 12), Xiawan (Ren 10), Neiguan (P 6), Gongsun (Sp 4)
D: Zhongwan (Ren 12), Zusanli (S 36), Sanyinjiao (Sp 6), Tianshu (S 25)
E: Neiguan (P 6), Gongsun (Sp 4), Jinjin (Extra), Yuye (Extra)

72. Which of the following points are the most commonly used ones for the treatment of hiccups? ( )

A: Zusanli (S 36) and Sanyinjiao (Sp 6)
B: Zhongwan (Ren 12) and Tianshu (S 25)
C: Geshu (B 17) and Neiguan (P 6)
D: Pishu (B 20) and Weishu (B 21)
E: Tanzhong (Ren 17) and Taichong (Liv 3)

73. Geshu (B 17) is utilized in the treatment of hiccups because ( ).

A: it is a point on the bladder channel
B: it is a Back-Shu point
C: it is one of the eight influential points
D: it has the function of regulating the blood
E: it is able to stop the Qi from ascending

74. Apart from the principal points such as Geshu (B 17), Neiguan (P 6) and Zhongwan (Ren 12), which of the following points would you select as supplementary points to treat hiccups caused by the stagnation of Qi? ( )

A: Tanzhong (Ren 17) and Taichong (Liv 3)
B: Juque (Ren 14) and Inner-Neiting (Extra)
C: Shangwan (Ren 13) and Zusanli (S 36)
D: Rugen (S 18) and Ganshu (B 18)
E:Sanyinjiao (Sp 6) and Hegu (LI 4)

75. The best prescription for the treatment of acute diarrhea is ( ).

A: Tianshu (S 25), Zhongwan (Ren 12), Zusanli (S 36), Yinlingquan (Sp 9)
B: Pishu (B 20), Zhongwan (Ren 12), Zhangmen (Liv 13), Zusanli (S 36)
C: Zusanli (S 36), Tianshu (S 25), Mingmen (Du 4), Guanyuan (Ren 4)
D: Pishu (B 20), Shenshu (B 23), Zhangmen (Liv 13), Mingmen (Du 4)
E: Taixi (K 3), Shenshu (B 23), Zusanli (S 36), Tianshu (S 25)

76. The basic points for the treatment of dysentery are ( ).

A: Zusanli (S 36) and Sanyinjiao (Sp 6)
B: Tianshu (S 25) and Shangjuxu (S 37)

C: Quchi (LI 11) and Hegu (LI 4)
D: Zhongwan (Ren 12) and Yinlingquan (Sp 9)
E: Neiguan (P 6) and Gongsun (P 4)

77. Tianshu (S 25), Shangjuxu (S 37), Zhongwan (Ren 12) and Neiguan (P 6) are the best presription for the treatment of ( ).

A: damp-heat dysentery
B: cold-damp dysentery
C: food-resistant dysentery
D: intermittent dysentery
E: none of the above

78. The prescription of Tianshu (S 25), Shangjuxu (S 37), Pishu (B 20), Weishu (B 21), Guanyuan (Ren 4), and Zusanli (S 36) is commonly used to treat ( ).

A: damp-heat dysentery
B: cold-damp dysentery
C: food-resistant dysentery
D: intermittent dysentery
E: none of the above

79. All the following points are main points for the treatment of abdominal distention except ( ).

A: Zhongwan (Ren 12)
B: Tianshu (S 25)
C: Zusanli (S 36)
D: Sanyinjiao (Sp 6)
E: Shangjuxu (S 37)

80. Zhongwan (Ren 12) combined with Zusanli (S 36) and Tianshu (S 25) combined with Shangjuxu (S 37) are both combinations of ( ).

A: Back-Shu point and Front-Mu point
B: Front-Mu point and Lower He-sea point
C: Yuan-Primary point and Luo-Connecting point
D: "mother" point and "son" point
E: none of the above

81. Which of the following prescriptions is the best one for a patient with the following signs and symptoms: abdominal distention relieved by pressure, borborygmus, loose stools, loss of appetite, lassitude, listlessness, a pale tongue with a white coating, and a forceless pulse? ( )

A: Hegu (LI 4), Tianshu (S 25), Zhongwan (Ren 12), Shangjuxu (S 37)

B: Hegu (LI 4), Qihai (Ren 6), Tianshu (S 25), Yinlingquan (Sp 9)
C: Guanyuan (Ren 4), Taibai (Sp 3), Zhongwan (Ren 12), Zusanli (S 36)
D: Pishu (B 20), Weishu (B 21), Tianshu (S 25), Liangqiu (S 34)
E: Guanyuan (Ren 4), Mingmen (Du 4), Shenque (Ren 8), Shenshu (B 23)

82. All the following points are main points for the treatment of prolapse of the rectum except ( ).

A: Baihui (Du 20)
B: Dachangshu (B 25)
C: Changqiang (Du 1)
D: Hegu (LI 4)
E: Zusanli (S 36)

83. Which of the following channels has points commonly selected to treat prolapse of the rectum? ( )

A: Ren channel
B: Du channel
C: slpeen channel
D: large intestine channel
E: stomach channel

84. All the following can cause edema except ( ).

A: invasion of the wind upon the lung
B: invasion of the dampness which affects the function of the spleen
C: sinking of spleen and stomach Qi
D: weakness of kidney Qi
E: weakness of spleen Qi

85. Which of the following points is commonly used as a supplementary point to treat facial puffiness? ( )

A: Shuigou (Du 26)
B: Jingming (B 1)
C: Ermen (SJ 21)
D: Daying (S 5)
E: Yingxiang (LI 20)

86. Which of the following prescriptions owuld be your first choice to treat a patient complaining of nocturnal enuresis? ( )

A: Pishu (B 20), Shenshu (B 23), Shuifen (Ren 9), Guanyuan (Ren 4)
B: Shenshu (B 23), Pangguangshu (B 28), Zhongji (Ren 3), Sanyinjiao

(Sp 6)
C: Fuliu (K 7), Taixi (K 3), Shenshu (B 23), Pangguangshu (B 28)
D: Lieque (L 7), Feishu (B 13), Hegu (LI 4), Weiyang (B 39)
E: Pishu (B 20), Yinlingquan (Sp 9), Sanyinjiao (Sp 6), Zusanli (S 36)

87. Which of the following prescriptions is the best to treat yang-edema? ( )
A: Pishu (B 20), Shenshu (B 23), Shuifen (Ren 9), Guanyuan (Ren 4)
B: Lieque (L 7), Hegu (LI 4), Pianli (LI 6), Weiyang (B 39)
C: Zhongji (Ren 3), Guanyuan (Ren 4), Qihai (Ren 6), Shenshu (B 23)
D: Zulinqi (G 41), Shangqiu (Sp 5), Pangguangshu (B 28), Zhongji (Ren 3)
E: Pishu (B 20), Sanyinjiao (Sp 6), Yinlingquan (Sp 9), Zusanli (S 36)

88. Which of the following points are commonly used as the supplementary points to treat edema of the dorsum pedis? ( )
A: Taixi (K 3) and Fuliu (K 7)
B: Jiaoxin (K 8) and Rangu (K 2)
C: Zulinqi (G 41) and Shangqiu (Sp 5)
D: Yinbai (Sp 1) and Taibai (Sp 3)
E: Lougu (Sp 7) and Diji (Sp 8)

89. The prescription of choice for the treatment of dysuria is ( ).
A: Sanyinjiao (Sp 6), Yinlingquan (Sp 9) and Diji (Sp 8)
B: Neiguan (P 6), Gongsun (Sp 4) and Sanyinjiao (Sp 6)
C: Pishu (B 20), Shenshu (B 23) and Sanyinjiao (Sp 6)
D: Shenshu (B 23), Zhongji (Ren 6) and Guanyuan (Ren 4)
E: Pangguangshu (B 28), Zhongji (Ren 3) and Yinlingquan (Sp 9)

90. Apart from the main points such as Pangguangshu (B 28) and Zhongji (Ren 3), which of the following points would you use as the supplementary points to treat dysuria with cloudy urine? ( )
A: Weiyang (B 39) and Shenmai (B 62)
B: Qihai (Ren 6) and Zusanli (S 36)
C: Xuehai (Sp 10) and Sanyinjiao (Sp 6)
D: Gongsun (Sp 4) and Yinbai (Sp 1)
E: Shenshu (B 23) and Zhaohai (K 6)

91. All the following points are commonly used to treat retention of urine caused by the accumulation of heat in the bladder except ( ).
A: Pangguangshu (B 28)
B: Zhongji (Ren 3)

C: Yinlingquan (Sp 9)
D: Weiyang (B 39)
E: Zhongwan (Ren 12)

92. All the following points are commonly used to treat impotence caused by the decline of Mingmen fire except ( ).

A: Yinlingquan (Sp 9)
B: Guanyuan (Ren 4)
C: Mingmen (DU 4)
D: Shenshu (B 23)
E: Taixi (K 3)

93. Which of the following prescriptions is the best for a male patient with the following signs and symptoms: impotence, bitter taste in the mouth, thirst, burning and dark red urine, a yellow, sticky tongue coating, and a soft, rapid pulse? ( )

A: Guanyuan (Ren 4), Mingmen (Du 4), Shenshu (B 23), Taixi (K 3)
B: Zhongji (Ren 3), Sanyinjiao (Sp 6), Yinlingquan (Sp 9), Zusanli (S 36)
C: Xinshu (B 15), Shenmen (H 7), Sanyinjiao (Sp 9), Zusanli (S 36)
D: Ganshu (B 18), Taichong (Liv 3), Xingjian (Liv 2), Neiting (S 44)
E: Zhongji (Ren 3), Guanyuan (Ren 4), Qihai (Ren 6), Shenshu (B 23)

94. Which of the following prescriptions is commonly selected to treat insomnia by the method of tapping-needling? ( )

A: Shenmen (H 7), Sanyinjiao (Sp 6) and Anmian (Extra)
B: Taixi (K 3) and Yinbai (Sp 1)
C: Sanyinjiao (Sp 6) and Zusanli (S 36)
D: Sishencong (Extra) and Huatuojiaji (Extra)
E: Wangu (G 12) and Neiguan (P 6)

95. Apart from the principal points such as Baihui (Du 20), Changqiang (Du 1) and Dachangshu (B 25), another point used to treat prolapse of the rectum is ( ).

A: Baihuanshu (B 30)
B: Tanzhong (Ren 17)
C: Erbai (Extra)
D: Chengshan (B 57)
E: none of the above

96. Apart from Dachangshu (B 25), Tianshu (S 25) and Zhigou (SJ 6), which of the following points would you select to treat constipation due to the

stagnation of Qi? ( )

A: Hegu (LI 4) and Quchi (LI 11)
B: Zhongwan (Ren 12) and Taichong (Liv 3)
C: Pishu (B 20) and Taichong (Liv 3)
D: Qihai (Ren 6) and Shenque (Ren 8)
E: Mingmen (Du 4) and Guanyuan (Ren 4)

97. The prescription formed by Shenmen (H 7), Sanyinjiao (Sp 6), Zusanli (S 36) and Xinshu (B 15) is used to treat insomnia caused by ( ).

A: dysfunction of the stomach
B: disharmony between the heart and kidney
C: upward disturbance of the liver fire
D: deficiency of the heart and spleen
E: deficiency of the heart and gallbladder

98. The best prescription selected in treatment of mental depression is ( ).

A: Xinshu (B 15), Ganshu (B 18), Pishu (B 20), Shenmen (H 7), Fenglong (S 40)
B: Dazhui (Du 14), Shuigou (Du 26), Fengfu (Du 16), Neiguan (P 6), Fenglong (S 40)
C: Pishu (B 20), Shenshu (B 23), Guanyuan (Ren 4), Zusanli (S 36)
D: Fengchi (G 20), Ganshu (B 18), Shenshu (B 23), Xingjian (Liv 2), Xiaxi (G 43)
E: Zhongwan (Ren 12), Neiguan (P 6), Fenglong (S 40), Jiexi (S 41)

99. Which of the following prescriptions is best indicated in mental disorders? ( )

A: Jiuwei (Ren 15), Dazhui (Du 14), Jianshi (P 5), Fenglong (S 40)
B: Dazhui (Du 14), Fengfu (Du 16), Shuigou (Du 26), Neiguan (P 6), Fenglong (S 40)
C: Fengchi (G 20), Shenshu (B 23), Guanyuan (Ren 4), Zusanli (S 36)
D: Ganshu (B 18), Xingjian (Liv 2), Neiguan (P 6), Xiaxi (G 43), Shenshu (B 23)
E: Zhongwan (Ren 12), Neiguan (P 6), Zusanli (S 36), Jiexi (S 41)

100. According to *Chinese Acupuncture and Moxibustion* besides the points Tiantu (Ren 22), Tanzhong (Ren 17) and Fenglong (S 40), which of the following points would you select to treat globus hysteircus? ( )

A: Shangwan (Ren 13) and Zhigou (SJ 6)

B; Ganshu (B 18) and Danshu (B 19)
C: Neiguan (P 6) and Taichong (Liv 3)
D: Zhongwan (Ren 12) and Zusanli (S 36)
E: Shenmen (H 7) and Juque (Ren 14)

101. All the following points are the main points for treatment of hysteria due to insufficiency of blood except ( ).

A: Juque (Ren 14)
B: Shenmen (H 7)
C: Sanyinjiao (Sp 6)
D: Taichong (Liv 3)
E: Fenglong (S 40)

102. Which of the following points can be used as the supplementary points to treat hysteria with sudden aphonia? ( )

A: Tongli (H 5) and Lianquan (Ren 23)
B: Neiguan (P 6) and Tanzhong (Ren 17)
C: Qihai (Ren 6) and Guanyuan (Ren 4)
D: Hegu (LI 4) and Yanglingquan (G 34)
E: Shuigou (Du 26) and Yongquan (K 1)

103. Which of the following points can be used as supplementary points to treat hysteria with hiccup? ( )

A: Tongli (H 5) and Lianquan (Ren 23)
B: Gongsun (Sp 4) and Tiantu (Ren 22)
C: Hegu (LI 4) and Yanglingquan (G 34)
D: Shuigou (Du 26) and Yongquan (K 1)
E: Neiguan (P 6) and Tanzhong (Ren 17)

104. Which of the following points have been proved effective in resuscitation? ( )

A: Tongli (H 5) and Lianquan (Ren 23)
B: Gongsun (Sp 4) and Tiantu (Ren 22)
C: Shuigou (Renzhong) (Du 26) and Yongquan (K 1)
D: Hegu (LI 4) and Yanglingquan (G 34)
E: Qihai (Ren 6) and Guanyuan (Ren 4)

105. All the following points may be selected in the treatment of temporal headache except ( ).

A: Taiyan (Extra)
B: Shuaigu (G 8)

C: Waiguan (SJ 5)
D: Zulinqi (G 41)
E: Houxi (SI 3)

106. All the following points are usually used for the treatment of parietal headache except ( ).

A: Baihui (Du 20)
B: Houxi (SI 3)
C: Zhiyin (B 67)
D: Zulinqi (G 41)
E: Taichong (Liv 3)

107. All the following points are commonly used to treat occipital headache due to the invasion of pathogenic wind except ( ).

A: Kunlun (B 60)
B: Neiting (S 44)
C: Houxi (SI 3)
D: Fengchi (G 20)
E: Fengfu (Du 16)

108. All the following points are commonly used to treat frontal headache except ( ).

A: Touwei (S 8)
B: Yintang (Extra)
C: Waiguan (SJ 5)
D: Hegu (LI 4)
E: Neiting (S 44)

109. All the following points are commonly used to treat pain in the supraorbital region except ( ).

A: Hegu (LI 4)
B: Yangbai (G 14)
C: Taiyang (Extra)
D: Zanzhu (B 2)
E: Waiguan (SJ 5)

110. All the following points are commonly used to treat pain at the mandibular region except ( ).

A: Xiaguan (S 7)
B: Jiache (S 6)
C: Hegu (LI 4)

D: Jiachengjiang (Extra)
E: Yingxiang (LI 20)

111. All the following points are commonly used to treat pain at the maxillary region except ( ).
A: Sibai (S 2)
B: Quanliao (SI 18)
C: Yingxiang (LI 20)
D: Yangbai (G 14)
E: Hegu (LI 4)

112. The prescription composed of Qimen (Liv 14), Zhigou (SJ 6), Yanglingquan (G 34), Geshu (B 17) and Ganshu (B 18) is best indicated if pain is in the hypochondriac region due to ( ).
A: stagnation of Qi
B: deficiency of the liver blood
C: stagnation of blood
D: retention of phlegm
E: none of the above

113. Apart from the main points, which of the following points are usually used as the supplementary points to treat Wandering-Bi syndromes? ( )
A: Geshu (B 17) and Xuehai (Sp 10)
B: Shenshu (B 23) and Guanyuan (Ren 4)
C: Zusanli (S 36) and Shangqiu (Sp 5)
D: Fengchi (GB 20) and Taiyang (Extra)
E: Dazhui (Du 14) and Quchi (LI 11)

114. Apart from the main points, which of the following points are usually used as the supplementary points to treat tendon-Bi syndromes? ( )
A: Dashu (B 11)
B: Quchi (LI 11)
C: Xuanzhong (G 39)
D: Xuehai (SP 10)
E: Yanglingquan (G 34)

115. In addition to the main points, which of the following points would you use first as supplementary points for a patient who complains of soreness, heaviness and pain of the joints which fail to perform their functions of lifting, extension and flexion? ( )
A: Geshu (B 17) and Xuehai (Sp 10)

B: Shenshu (B 23) and Guanyuan (Ren 4)
C: Dashu (B 11) and Xuanzhong (G 39)
D: Quchi (LI 11) and Yanglingquan (G 34)
E: Zusanli (S 36) and Shangqiu (Sp 5)

116. In addition to the local points, which of the following points would you select to treat heat-Bi syndromes? (   )

A: Geshu (B 17) and Tanzhong (Ren 17)
B: Dazhui (Du 14) and Quchi (LI 11)
C: Dashu (B 11) and Xuanzhong (G 39)
D: Zusanli (S 36) and Sanyinjiao (Sp 6)
E: Yanglingquan (G 34) and Taichong (Liv 3)

117. Which of the following points are best indicated in Wei-syndromes due to heat in the lung? (   )

A: Yuji (L 10) and Kongzui (L 6)
B: Feishu (B 13) and Chize (L 5)
C: Lieque (L 7) and Hegu (LI 4)
D: Shaochang (L 11) and Erjian (LI 2)
E: none of the above

118. The prescription composed of Zhongji (Ren 3), Xuehai (Sp 10), Taichong (Liv 3), Hegu (LI 4) and Sanyinjiao (Sp 6) is indicated in (   ).

A: dysmenorrhea of the deficiency type
B: antedated menstruation
C: irregular menstrual cycles
D: amenorrhea due to blood deficiency
E: amenorrhea due to blood stagnation

119. Amenorrhea due to blood deficiency is treated by the prescription composed of (   ).

A: Ganshu (B 18), Pishu (B 20), Shenshu (B 23), Zusanli (S 36) and Guanyuan (Ren 4)
B: Zhongji (Ren 3), Guilai (S 29), Hegu (LI 4), Xuehai (Sp 10) and Sanyinjiao (Sp 6)
C: Xuehai (Sp 10), Geshu (B 17), Taichong (Liv 3), Xingjian (Liv 2) and Zusanli (S 36)
D: Pishu (B 20), Mingmen (Du 4), Guanyuan (Ren 4), Sanyinjiao (Sp 3) and Diji (Sp 8)
E: none of the above

120. A patient has the following signs and symptoms: profuse, thin and light-red menses with a shortened cycle, lassitude, empty and heavy sensations in the lower abdomen (no findings of this, just the patient's subjective sensations), pale tongue with thin coating, and a weak pulse. The prescription used for this patient should be ( ).

A: Quchi (LI 11), Zhongji (Ren 3), Xuehai (Sp 10) and Shuiquan (K 5)
B: Qihai (Ren 6), Sanyinjiao (Sp 6), Zhongwan (Ren 12) and Zusanli (S 36)
C: Xuehai (Sp 10), Jiaoxin (K 8), Sanyinjiao (Sp 6) and Guilai (S 29)
D: Taichong (Liv 3), Taixi (L 3), Sanyinjiao (Sp 6) and Xingjian (Liv 3)
E: none of the above

121. Which of the following points is used as the supplementary one to treat ant edated menstruation due to heat in the blood caused by deficient yin? ( )

A: Hegu (LI 4)
B: Xinjian (Liv 2)
C: Rangu (K 2)
D: Neiting (S 44)
E: none of the above

122. In addition to the main points which of the following points is also used to treat antedated menstruation due to heat in the blood transformed from stagnated liver Qi? ( )

A: Rangu (K 2)
B: Neiting (S 44)
C: Ganshu (B 18)
D: Xinjian (Liv 2)
E: none of the above

123. In dealing with a malpositioned fetus, which of the following points should you utilize to correct the position? ( )

A: Diji (Sp 8)
B: Sanyinjiao (Sp 6)
C: Taixi (K 3)
D: Shangqiu (S 5)
E: Zhiyin (B 67)

124. Which of the following points are commonly used for prolonged labour? ( )

A: Taichong (Liv 3) and Neiguan (P 6)

B: Guanyuan and Shenshu (B 23)
C: Qihai (Ren 6) and Zusanli (S 36)
D: Sanyinjiao (Sp 6) and Zhiyin (B 67)
E: none of the above

125. The best prescription for insufficient lactation is ( ).

A: Tanzhong (Ren 17) and Shaoze (SI 1)
B: Tanzhong (Ren 17) and Zusanli (S 36)
C: Zulinqi (B 41) and Hegu (LI 4)
D: Hegu (LI 4) and Zusanli (S 36)
E: Guangming (B 37) and Zulinqi (B 41)

126. Which of the following points is an effective and empirical lactogenic point? ( )

A: Tanzhong (Ren 17)
B: Rugen (S 18)
C: Shaochong (H 9)
D: Shaoze (SI 1)
E: Sanyinjiao (Sp 6)

127. For the treatment of mumps, moxibustion with medulla junci can be used on ( ).

A: Jiaosun (SJ 20)
B: Jiache (S 6)
C: Yifeng (SJ 17)
D: Taichong (Liv 3)
E: Hegu (LI 4)

128. For the treatment of torticollis, which of the following points is added for difficulty in rotating the neck?( )

A: Feishu (B 13)
B: Zhizheng (SI 7)
C: Lieque (L 7)
D: Hegu (LI 4)
E: Kongzui (L 6)

129. For the treatment of torticollis, which of the following points are added for inability of flexion and extension? ( )

A: Kunlun (B 60) and Lieque (L 7)
B: Zhizheng (SI 7) and Kongzui (L 6)
C: Hegu (LI 4) and Chize (L 5)

D: Taiyuan (L 9) and Yifeng (SJ 17)
E: none of the above

130. All the following points are commonly used to treat a stiff neck except ( ).
A: Tianzhu (B 10)
B: Jianwaishu (SI 14)
C: Xuanzhong (G 39)
D: Houxi (SI 3)
E: Yifeng (SJ 17)

131. All the following points are commonly used to treat tinnitus except ( ).
A: Houxi (SI 3)
B: Yifeng (SJ 17)
C: Tinghui (G 2)
D: Xiaxi (G 34)
E: Zhongzhu (SJ 3)

132. All the following points are commonly used to treat epistaxis due to deficiency of yin with preponderance of fire except ( ).
A: Yingxiang (LI 20)
B: Shaoshang (L 11)
C: Hegu (LI 4)
D: Shangxing (Du 23)
E: Zhaohai (K 6)

133. All the following points are commonly used to treat toothache due to stomach fire except ( ).
A: Hegu (LI 4)
B: Jiache (S 6)
C: Neiting (S 44)
D: Xiaguan (S 7)
E: Fengchi (G 20)

134. In addition to local points, which of the following points would you select to treat a toothache caused by deficiency of kidney fire? ( )
A: Yongquan (K 1)
B: Rangu (K 2)
C: Taixi (K 3)
D: Dazhong (K 4)
E: Shuiquan (K 5)

135. Which of the following channels has points usually selected to treat

toothache caused by wind-fire? ( )

A: Hand-Shaoyang channel
B: Hand-Yangming channel
C: Foot-Shaoyang channel
D: Foot-yangming channel
E: none of the above

136. Which of the following points can be used by the pricking method to treat sore throat? ( )

A: Yuji (L 10)
B: Shaoshang (L 11)
C: Hegu (LI 4)
D: Neiting (S 44)
E: Tianrong (SI 17)

137. The prescription composed of Jiache (S 6), Xiaguan (S 7) and Taixi (K 3) is used to treat ( ).

A: toothache due to stomach fire
B: toothache caused by wind fire
C: toothache caused by deficiency of kidney yin
D: sore throat due to an excess of heat
E: sore throat due to yin deficiency

138. The prescription composed of Jingming (B 1), Fengchi (G 20), Taiyang (Extra), Hegu (LI 4) and Xingjian (Liv 2) is used to treat ( ).

A: epistaxis
B: nasal obstruction
C:deafness and tinnitus
D: congestion, swelling and pain of the eye
E: toothache

139. For the treatment of urticaria, which of the following pairs of points can be used to eliminate heat in the blood? ( )

A: Quchi (LI 11) and Hegu (LI 4)
B: Xuehai (Sp 10) and Weizhong (B 40)
C: Taichong (Liv 3) and Neiting (S 44)
D: Xingjian (Liv 2) and Sanyinjiao (Sp 6)
E: Hegu (LI 4) and Neiguan (P 6)

140. A patient has the following signs and symptoms: profuse and continuous vaginal discharge, soreness of the lower back, a cold sensation in the

lower abdomen , frequent and excessive urine, loose stools, a pale tongue with a thin coating, and a deep pulse. Which of the following prescriptions would you select for this patient? (   )

A: Shenshu (B 23), Guanyuan (Ren 4) Dahe (K 12), Daimai (G 26), Fuliu (K 7)

B: Zhongji (Ren 3), Ciliao (B 32), Sanyinjiao (Sp 6) and Taichong (Liv 3)

C: Daimai (B 26), Qihai (Ren 6) Baihuanshu (B 30), Yinlingquan (Sp 9) and Zusanli (S 36)

D: Shenshu (B 23), Pishu (B 20), Sanyinjiao (Sp 6), Yinlingquan (Sp 9) and Zusanli (S 36)

E: Ligou (Liv 5), Xuehai (Sp 10), Quchi (LI 11) and Neiting (S 44)

141. All the following points are principal points for the treatment of breast abscess except (   ).

A: Jianjing (G 21)

B: Shaoze (SI 1)

C: Rugen (S 18)

D: Tanzhong (Ren 17)

E: Shaoshang (L 11)

142. All the following points are commonly used to treat appendicitis except (   ).

A: Qihai (Ren 6)

B: Tianshu (S 25)

C: Quchi (LI 11)

D: Lanwei (Extra)

E: Shangjuxu (S 37)

143. A male patient has the following signs and symptoms: hypochondriac pain accompanied by heaviness of the body, and a sticky white tongue coating. According to the differentiation of syndromes of the channels, the prescription of choice at this stage is (   ).

A: Neiguan (LP 6) and Tianchi (P 1)

B: Zhigou (SJ 6) and Ahshi point (Extra)

C: Yanglingquan (GB 34) and Riyue (GB 24)

D: Taichong (Liv 3) and Qimen (Liv 14)

E: Taibai (Sp 3) and Dabao (Sp 21)

144. Which of the following procedures is most appropriate for treating painful Bi (obstruction) syndrome? (   )

A: Reinforcing manipulation together with moxibustion

B: Even movement together with moxibustion
C: Proper insertion with needle retention and moxibustion
D: Swift insertion and withdrawal
E: Bloodletting at the 12 Jing-Well points

145. After previous acupuncture treatments, a patient's hearing has improved but alalia remains. Which of the following points would you add at this time? ( )

A: Fengchi (GB 20) and Fengfu (Du 16)
B: Fengchi (GB 20) and Quchi (LI 11)
C: Quchi (LI 11) and Waiguan (SJ 5)
D: Waiguan (SJ 5) and Hegu (LI 4)
E: Hegu (LI 4) and Dazhui (Du 14)

146. Which of the following auricular acu-points is most likely employed to treat fever, hypertension and inflammation? ( )

A: blood pressure reducing groove
B: hypertension point
C: ear apex
D: Shenmen point
E: adrenal gland point

147. In dealing with disorders of the upper limbs, which prescription is the best selection? ( )

A: Huatuojiaji points vertebrae C1-3
B: Huatuojiaji points vertebrae C2-5
C: Huatuojiaji points vertebrae C3-T1
D: Huatuojiaji points vertebrae C6-T10
E: none of the above

148. The best prescription for treating insufficient lactation and tenderness of the breasts is ( )

A: Tanzhong (Ren 17), Rugen (St 10), Shaochong (H 9)
B: Zhongwan (Ren 12), Rugen (St 10), Shaoze (SI 1)
C: Qimen (Liv 14), Zhangmen (Liv 13), Zusanli (St 36)
D: Tanzhong (Ren 17), Rugen (St 10), Shaoze (SI 1)
E: Qimen (Liv 14), Tanzhong (Ren 17), Zusanli (St 36)

149. In which period during pregnancy is moxibustion most effective to correct the position of the fetus? ( )

A: After eight months of pregnancy

B: After seven months of pregnancy
C: After six months of pregnancy
D: After five months of pregnancy
E: After four months of pregnancy

150. A trigeminal neuralgia patient suddenly experiences dizziness, nausea, pallor and weak pulse after receiving needling at the point Hegu (LI 4). The appropriate initial management should be ( ).

A: Withdraw the needle and let the patient lay on his/her back
B: Puncture the points Shuigou (Du 26), Neiguan (P 6) and Zusanli (St 36)
C: Apply acupuncture and moxibustion to the points Baihui (Du 20) and Qihai (Ren 6)
D: Apply moxibustion to the points Shenque (Ren 8) and Zusanli (St 36)
E: All of the above

151. With a patient who has vomitting and diarrhea of the cold deficiency type, which one of the following indirect moxibustion techniques is indicated? ( )

A: moxibustion on salt
B: Moxibustion on ginger
C; Warm needle moxibustion
D: all of the above
E: none of the above

152. Using a three-edged needle is indicated in the following cases ( ).

A: lumbago due to stagnation of blood
B; high fever
C: sour throat
D: all of the above
E: none of the above

153. A young patient has the following signs and symptoms: heavy and aching sensation of the body, lassitude and shortness of breath following walking. Which of the following points would you use as the main point for treatment? ( )

A: Zusanli (S 36)
B: Yinlinquan (GB 34)
C: Zhangmen (Liv 13)
D: Dabao (Sp 21)
E: Tanzhong (Ren 17)

154. A patient has asthma plus the following signs and symptoms: short and

rapid breathing, weak voice, hidrosis and weak pulse. The points that would be best are ( ).

A: Qihai (Ren 6), Shenshu (UB 23)
B: Zusanli (St 36), Tanzhong (Ren 17)
C: Feishu (UB 13), Gaohuangshu (UB 43)
D: Tiantu (Ren 22), Pingchuan (Extra)
E: none of the above

155. In treating neurodermatitis the most likely used needle is ( ).

A: three-edged needle
B: cutaneous needle
C: intradermal needle
D: ordinary needle
E: none of the above

156. Cough with a small amount of sputum, or blood-tinged sputum, dryness of the mouth and throat, soreness and weakness of the lumbar region and knee joints, tidal fever, malar flush, night sweating, nocturnal emission, a red tongue with little coating and a thready, rapid pulse (*xi* and *shuo mai*) indicates ( ).

A: deficiency of the lung and kidney yin
B: deficiency of the lung and kidney Qi
C: imbalance between the liver and spleen
D: invasion of the lung and liver by fire
E: none of the above

157. Asthmatic breathing, shortness of breath and more exhalation than inhalation which are all exacerbated upon exertion, as well as a low voice, cold limbs, bluish complexion, spontaneous sweating, incontinence of urine due to severe cough, a pale tongue with a thin coating and a weak pulse (*ruo mai*) indicates ( ).

A: deficiency of heart Qi
B: deficiency of lung and kidney Qi
C: deficiency of spleen and lung Qi
D: deficiency of spleen and kidney yang
E: none of the above

158. Dizziness, blurred vision, dryness of the throat, tinnitus, heat sensations in the chest, palms and soles, soreness and weakness of the lumbar region and knee joints, malar flush, night sweating, nocturnal emissions, scanty menstrual flow, a red tongue with little coating and a thready, rapid

pulse (*xi* and *shuo mai*) indicates ( ).

A: deficiency of lung and kidney yin
B: deficiency of liver and kidney yin
C: deficiency of heart yin
D: disharmony between the heart and kidney
E: disharmony between the liver and spleen

159. Pallor, cold limbs, soreness and weakness of the lumbar region, diarrhea at dawn, facial puffiness, edema of the limbs, a pale, swollen and delicate tongue with a thin white coating and a deep weak pulse (*chen* and *ruo mai*) indicate ( ).

A: deficiency of spleen and kidney yang
B: deficiency of lung and kidney yin
C: deficiency of lung and kidney Qi
D: invasion of the spleen by cold-damp
E: deficiency of spleen yang

160. General lassitude, cough with profuse, dilute and white sputum, poor appetite, loose stools, a pale tongue with white coating and a weak pulse (*ruo mai*) in dicates a/an ( ).

A: deficiency of spleen and kidney yang
B: disharmony between the liver and stomach
C: deficiency of lung and spleen Qi
D: imbalance between the liver and spleen
E: none of the above

161. Distention, fullness and pain in the costal and hypochondriac regions, mental depression, poor appetite, abdominal distention, loose stools, a thin tongue coating and a string-taut (*xuan mai*) pulse indicate ( ).

A: deficiency of lung and kidney yin
B: deficiency of spleen and kidney yang
C: deficiency of liver and kidney yin
D: imbalance between the liver and spleen
E: deficiency of the spleen and stomach

162. Distention and pain in the costal, hypochondriac and epigastric regions, belching, acid regurgitation, an empty and uncomfortable sensation in the stomach, mental depression, a thin tongue coating and a string-taut pulse (*xuan mai*) indicate ( ).

A: deficiency of spleen and kidney yang

B: disharmony between the liver and the stomach
C: invasion of the lung by the liver
D: damp-heat in the middle Jiao
E: none of the above

163. The clinical manifestations of a sallow complexion, general lassitude, palpitation, poor memory, insomnia, dream-disturbed sleep, reduced appetite, abdominal distention, loose stools, a pale tongue with a thin, white coating and a thready weak pulse (*xi* and *ruo mai*) indicate ( ).

A: damp heat in the upper Jiao
B: disharmony between the heart and kidney
C: deficiency of both the heart and spleen
D: imbalance between the liver and spleen
E: deficiency of the spleen and stomach

Solutions to the Exercises

I.

1. E; 2. C; 3. D; 4. B; 5. A; 6. B; 7. C; 8. D; 9. A; 10. E; 11. C; 12. C; 13. A ; 14. B; 15. C; 16. D; 17. D; 18. E; 19. B; 20. B; 21. E; 22. B; 23. A; 24. E; 2 5. D; 26. D; 27. B; 28. A; 29. B; 30.C.

II.

1. C; 2. D; 3. B; 4. E; 5. A; 6. B; 7. C; 8. B; 9. D; 10. B; 11. C; 12. A; 13. C ; 14. D; 15. D; 16. D; 17. A; 18. C; 19. A; 20. B; 21. A; 22. B; 23. C; 24. B; 2 5. B; 26. E; 27. E; 28. E; 29. D; 30. C; 31. B; 32. C; 33. B; 34. D; 35. E; 36. C; 37. A; 38. D; 39. B; 40. A; 41. A; 42. C; 43. D; 44. B; 45. E; 46. C.

III.

1. B; 2. C; 3.E; 4. C; 5. D; 6. D; 7. A; 8. B; 9. C; 10. A; 11. C; 12. B; 13. D; 14. B; 15. A; 16. E; 17. B; 18. C; 19. A; 20. D; 21. C; 22. A; 23. A; 24. C; 25 . C; 26. D; 27. A; 28. B; 29. D; 30. D; 31. E; 32. D; 33. C; 34. A; 35. C; 36. C ; 37. D; 38. C; 39. E; 40. B; 41. C; 42. C; 43. A; 44. E; 45. B; 46. B; 47. B; 4 8. C; 49. E; 50. D; 51. C; 52. E; 53. C; 54. D; 55. C; 56. E; 57. B; 58. A; 59. D; 60. B; 61. C; 62. C; 63. C; 64. C; 65. A; 66. B; 67. A; 68. B; 69. D; 70. E; 71. B; 72. A; 73. A; 74. B; 75. D; 76. B; 77. B; 78. C; 79. E; 80. B; 81. B; 82. A; 83. C; 84. C; 85. C; 86. D; 87. E; 88. D; 89. D; 90. C; 91. C; 92. E; 93. A; 94. E; 95. B; 96. A; 97. D; 98. B; 99. A; 100. C; 101. B; 102. C; 103. C; 104. A; 105. A; 106. C; 107. D; 108. D; 109. D; 110. D; 111. E; 112. C; 113. C; 114. C; 115. D; 116. C; 117. E.

IV.

1. D; 2. B; 3. C;4. D; 5. A; 6. E; 7. B; 8. A; 9. C; 10. D; 11. B; 12. A; 13. E; 14. B; 15. D; 16. D; 17. C; 18. A; 19. C; 20. A; 21. C; 22. B; 23. A; 24. B; 25 . C; 26. A; 27. D; 28. A; 29. B; 30. C; 31. C; 32. D; 33. E; 34. C; 35. B; 36. A ; 37. A; 38. C; 39. B; 40. D; 41. A; 42. A; 43. B; 44. D; 45. C; 46. A; 47. A; 4 8. E; 49. D; 50. E; 51. C; 52. C; 53. C; 54. D.

V.

1. D; 2. C; 3. D; 4. A; 5. B; 6. C; 7. E; 8. B; 9. E; 10. A; 11. C; 12. E; 13. A ; 14. E; 15. C; 16. B; 17. D; 18. C; 19. B; 20. C; 21. A; 22. A; 23. D; 24. C; 2 5. B; 26. D; 27. B. B; 28. C; 29. E; 30. D; 31. E; 32. C; 33. D; 34. C; 35. B; 3 6. A; 37. A; 38. D; 39. A; 40. B; 41. E; 42. A; 43. C; 44. D; 45. E; 46. E; 47. B; 48. E; 49. E; 50. C; 51. E; 52. D; 53. A; 54. D; 55. C; 56. E; 57. E.

VI.

1. C; 2. A; 3. B; 4. C; 5. D; 6. B; 7. D; 8. E; 9. B; 10. C; 11. E; 12. C; 13. D ; 14. E; 15. A; 16. A; 17. E; 18. E; 19. B; 20. C; 21. C; 22. C; 23. E.

VII.

1. C; 2. A; 3. B; 4. D; 5. E; 6. E; 7. D; 8. C; 9. B; 10. E; 11. D; 12. C; 13. D ; 14. C; 15. A; 16. B; 17. C; 18. B; 19. B; 20. E; 21. C; 22. E; 23. A; 24. D; 2 5. C; 26. A; 27. C; 28. C; 29. B; 30. C; 31. B; 32. E; 33. C; 34. C; 35. A; 36. C; 37. C; 38. A; 39. B; 40. B; 41. E; 42. A; 43. B; 44. C; 45. D; 46. A; 47. C; 48. B; 49. D; 50. E; 51. A; 52. B; 53. D; 54. E; 55. B; 56. D; 57. C; 58. B; 59. A; 60. C; 61. D; 62. C; 63. B; 64. D; 65. E; 66. D; 67. B; 68. D; 69. D; 70. C; 71. A; 72. C; 73. E; 74. A; 75. A; 76. B; 77. C; 78. D; 79. D; 80. B; 81. C; 82 . D; 83. B; 84. C; 85. A; 86. B; 87. B; 88. C; 89. E; 90. E; 91. E; 92. A; 93. B ; 94. D; 95. E; 96. B; 97. D; 98. A; 99. B; 100. C; 101. E; 102. A; 103. B; 104. C; 105. E; 106. D; 107. B; 108. C; 109. A; 110. E; 111. D; 112. C; 113. A; 114. E; 115. C; 116. B; 117. B; 118. E; 119. A; 120. B; 121. C; 122. D; 123. E; 124. D; 125. A; 126. D; 127. A; 128. B; 129. A; 130. E; 131. A; 132. B; 133. E; 134. C; 135. A; 136. B; 137. C; 138. D; 139. B; 140. A; 141. E; 142. A; 143. D; 144. C; 145. D; 146. C; 147. A; 148. D; 149. B; 150. A; 151. B; 152. D; 153. D; 154. C; 155. B; 156. A; 157. B; 158. B; 159. A; 160. C; 161. D; 162. B; 163. C

"B" Type Questions

Each question contains a group of options that are followed by a series of questions. For EACH question in the series select the answer you consider to be correct. An answer may be chosen several times or not at all.

Example:
For each statement select the answer most closely associated with it.
A: Tanzhong (Ren 17)
B: Juque (Ren 14)
C: Shimen (Ren 5)
D: Guanyuan (Ren 4)
E: Zhongji (Ren 3)
Example 1. The Front-Mu point of the Sanjiao channel is ( ).
Example 2. The Front-Mu point of the small intestine channel is ( ).
Example 3. The Front-Mu point of the pericardium channel is ( ).
Example 4. The influential point of Qi is ( ).

The correct answers are C, D, A and A respectively and would be marked in the ( ).

Answers 1. C, 2. D, 3. A, 4. A.

I. Yin-Yang and the Five Elements

A: Wood
B: Metal
C: Water
D: Fire
E: Earth
1. The element of the Jing-River points on the yang channels is ( ).
2. The element of the Shu-Stream points on the yin channels is ( ).
3. The element of the Jing-Well points on the yang channels is ( ).
4. The element of the Jing-River points on the yin channels is ( ).

A: a weakness of yin leading to a preponderance of yang
B: a preponderance of yin consuming yang
C: a weakness of yang leading to a preponderance of yin
D: a preponderance of yang consuming yin
5. Cold syndrome of the Shi type may be caused by ( ).
6. Heat syndrome of the Shi type may be caused by ( ).
7. Cold syndrome of the Xu type may be caused by ( ).
8. Heat syndrome of the Xu type may be caused by ( ).

A: a disorder of "the son affecting the mother"
B: a disorder of "the mother affecting the son"
9. If the lung is affected by a disorder of the spleen, the disease is known as (   ).
10. If the lung is affected by a disorder of the kidney, the disease is referred to as (   ).

II. Zang-Fu, Qi, Blood and Body Fluid

A: controlling blood and vessels
B: storing blood
C: governing blood
D: receiving Qi
E: dominating Qi and controlling respiration
F: maintaining patency for the flow of Qi
G: controlling the tendons
H: dominating the hair and skin
I: dominating the muscles
J: dominating the bone
K: dominating the water metabolism
L: regulating water passages
M: governing transportation and transformation
1. The function(s) of the liver include(s) (   ).
2. The function(s) of the heart include(s) (   ).
3. The function(s) of the spleen include(s) (   ).
4. The function(s) of the lung include(s) (   ).
5. The function(s) of the kidney include(s) (   ).

A: a Zang organ
B: a Fu organ
C: an extraordinary organ
D: both a Fu organ and an extraordinary organ
6. The uterus is (   ).
7. The urinary bladder is (   ).
8. The brain is (   ).
9. The gallbladder is (   ).
10. The spleen is (   ).
11. Sanjiao is (   ).

Each Zang organ opens to a sense organ. This indicates the close structural or physiological relationship between the internal organs and the sense organs.

A: tongue
B: nose
C: ear
D: mouth
E: eye

12. The lung opens to the ( ).
13. The liver opens to the ( ).
14. The spleen opens to the ( ).
15. The heart opens to the ( ).
16. The kidney opens to the ( ).

A: liver
B: kidney
C: heart
D: pericardium
E: lung
F: spleen

17. The small intestine is externally-internally related with the ( ).
18. The large intestine is externally-internally related with the ( ).
19. The stomach is externally-internally related with the ( ).
20. The gallbladder is externally-internally related with the ( ).
21. The urinary bladder is externally-internally related with the ( ).
22. The Sanjiao is externally-internally related with the ( ).

A: is related to reproductive function
B: circulates in the vessels and supplies the viscera
C: circulates outside the vessels and is mainly distributed in the muscles and skin to warm and nourish the subcutaneous tissues
D: nourishes the heart and lung and promotes their functions of dominating blood and vessels and performing respiration

23. Essential Qi (Zong Qi) ( ).
24. Nutrient Qi (Ying Qi) ( ).
25. Defensive Qi (Wei (Qi) ( ).
26. Source Qi (Yuan Qi) ( ).

A: Yin
B: Yang

27. The Qi of the heart belongs to ( ).

28. Body fluid belongs to ( ).
29. Blood belongs to ( ).

A: to manufacture and store essential substances
B: to receive and digest food, absorb nutrient substances, and transmit and excrete wastes

30. The main function of the six Fu organs is ( ).
31. The main function of the five Zang organs is ( ).

III. The Channels, Collaterals and Acupoints

A: febrile disease
B: stifling sensation in the chest
C: nausea, diarrhea
D: cough, sore throat, aversion to cold
E: painful joints caused by exogenous wind and cold

1. The Jing-River points are often used to treat ( ).
2. The Shu-Stream points are often used to treat ( ).
3. The He-Sea points are often used to treat ( ).

A: Wangu (SI 4)
B: Shenmen (H 7)
C: Taixi (K 3)
D: Tongli (H 5)
E: Zhizheng (SI 7)

The following stem pertains to questions 4-5

A patient has the following signs and symptoms: insomnia, restlessness, flushed face, dry mouth, difficult urination, scanty in amount and red in colour, and burning pain in the urethra. In making a prescription according to the matching method of Yuan-Source and Lou-Connecting points, 4. the Yuan point used would be ( ), and 5. the Luo point used would be ( ).

A: the channel of Hand-Taiyang, the channel of Foot-Taiyang, the channel of Foot -Shaoyang
B: the channel of Hand-Taiyang, the channel of Foot-Shaoyang, the channel of Hand-Shaoyang
C: the channel of Hand-Taiyang, the channel of Foot-Shaoyang, the channel of Hand-Yangming
D: the channel of Hand-Taiyang, the channel of Foot-Yangming, the channel

of Hand-Jueyin

6. The channels with distribution to the centre of the ear include ( ).
7. The channels with distribution to or connected with the lung include ( ).

A: sympathetic
B: Shenmen
C: adrenal gland
D: subcortex
E: occiput

8. The auricular point used in treating mental disorders, skin diseases or syncope is ( ).
9. The auricular point effective in relieving symptoms of the digestive and circulatory systems is ( ).

A: diseases of the reproductive system
B: weak or no pulse
C: biliary ascariasis
D: diseases of the circulatory system
E: inflammation

10. The root of the ear vagus is indicated in ( ).
11. The endocrine point is indicated in ( ).
12. The sympathetic point is indicated in ( ).
13. The point adrenal gland is recommended for patients suffering from ( ).
14. The point subcortex is commonly employed to treat ( ).

A: Zulinqi (GB 41)
B: Jiaxi (GB 43)
C: Zuqiaoyin (GB 44)
D: Yangfu (GB 38)
E: Yanglingquan (GB 34)

15. The Jing-Well point of the gallbladder channel is ( ).
16. The Xing-Spring point of the gallbladder channel is ( ).
17. The Shu-Stream point of the gallbladder channel is ( ).
18. The Jing-River point of the gallbladder channel is ( ).
19. The He-sea point of the gallbladder channel is ( ).

A: Shangjuxu (St 37)
B: Zusanli (St 36)
C: Xiajuxu (St 39)
D: Yanglingquan (GB 34)

E: Weiyang (UB 39)
20. The lower He-Sea point of the Sanjiao is ( ).
21. The lower He-Sea point of the stomach is ( ).
22. The lower He-Sea point of the large intestine is ( ).
23. The lower He-Sea point of the small intestine is ( ).
24. The lower He-Sea point of the gallbladder is ( ).

A: Geshu (UB 17)
B: Yanglingquan (GB 34)
C: Dashu (UB 11)
25. The influential point for bones is ( ).
26. The influential point for blood is ( ).
27. The influential point for tendons and muscles is ( ).

A: Yuji (Lu 10)
B: Jingqu (Lu 8)
C: Kongzui (Lu 6)
D: Taiyuan (Lu 9)
E: Chize (Lu 5)
28. Xi-Cleft point(s) include(s) ( ).
29. Shu point(s) include(s) ( ).

A: 2 cun lateral to the midline at the level of the sternum
B: 4 cun lateral to the midline at the level of the sternum
C: 6 cun lateral to the midline at the level of the sternum
D: 2 cun lateral to the midline at the level of the abdomen
E: 0.5 cun lateral to the midline at the level of the abdomen
30. The course of the stomach channel runs ( ).
31. The course of the kidney channel runs ( ).
32. The course of the spleen channel runs ( ).

IV. Diagnostic Methods

A: pale complexion
B: red colour
C: malar flush
D: pale yellow complexion
E: bluish colour
1. Yin excess is reflected by ( ).

2. Stagnation is reflected by ( ).
3. Deficiency of both Qi and blood is reflected by ( ).

A: deficiency of the kidney
B: deficiency of Qi
C: dificiency of blood
D: deficiency of the spleen
E: deficiency of yin

4. A malar flush indicates ( )
5. A dark grey colour indicates ( ).

A: deficiency of Qi and excess of phlegm-dampness
B: deficiency of the kidney
C: insufficiency of blood
D: invasion of dampness
E: excessive heat

6. A thin person with dry skin suggests ( ).
7. An overweight person with mental depression suggests ( ).

A: yellow sclera
B: redness and swelling of the eye
C: flaring the flapping of the ala nasi
D: dry and withered auricles

8. Consumption of the kidney essence is suggested when there is ( ).
9. The fire causes ( )
10. Heat in the lung is suggested when there is ( ).

A: deficiency of blood
B: deficiency of Qi
C: flare-up of stomach fire
D: flare-up liver fire
E: disturbance of liver wind

11. Redness and swelling of the gums are due to ( ).
12. Pale gums suggest ( ).
13. Deviation of the mouth and eye is often caused by ( ).

A: the tip of the tongue
B: the central part of the tongue
C: the border of the tongue
D: the root (posterior) of the tongue
E: the surface of the tongue

14. The pathological changes of the kidney are revealed on ( ).
15. The pathological changes of the heart and lung are revealed on ( ).
16. The pathological changes of the spleen and stomach are revealed on ( ).

A: thick coating
B: moist coating
C: sticky coating
D: peeled coating
E: dry coating

17. The consumption of Qi and yin of the stomach presents ( ).
18. invasion of the damp is suggested by ( ).

A: deficiency of blood
B: deficiency of yin
C: stagnation of blood
D: excess heat
E: stagnation of Qi

19. A pale tongue suggests ( ).
20. A blue purple tongue suggests ( ).

A: consumption of Qi and yin of the stomach
B: invasion of damp-heat in the interior
C: consumption of the kidney essence
D: hyperactivity of the fire due to deficiency of yin
E: consumption of body fluid due to extreme heat

21. A red tongue with a black dry coating indicates ( ).
22. A red tongue with a yellow, sticky coating indicates ( ).
23. A thin red tongue with a thin, dry coating indicates ( ).

A: a red tongue with a thick, yellow coating
B: a pale tongue witha white, moist coating
C: a red tongue with a yellow, sticky coating
D: a slightly red tongue with a thin, white coating
E: a deep-red tongue with little coating

24. The syndrome of hyperactivity of the fire due to deficiency of yin is suggested by ( ).
25. The syndrome of excess heat is suggested by ( ).
26. The syndrome of deficient cold reveals ( ).

A: excessive heat and the consuming body fluids
B: deficiency of blood

C: retention of phlegm
D: retention of food
E: winstroke

27. A red, cracked tongue suggests ( ).
28. A pale, cracked tongue suggests ( ).
29. A tongue deviated to one side suggests ( ).

A: deficiency of yin
B: retention of dampness
C: excess heat in the Yangming channel
D: intermediate syndromes
E: exterior syndromes

30. Afternoon fever with constipation and fullness and pain in the abdomen suggests ( ).
31. Chills accompanied by fever suggests ( ).
32. Alternating chills and fever suggests ( ).

A: distending pain
B: pricking pain
C: pain with a heavy sensation
D: colicky pain
E: burning sensation

33. Heat syndromes often manifests ( ).
34. Stagnation of blood often causes ( ).
35. Invasion of dampness often manifests ( ).
36. Stagnation of Qi often causes ( ).

A: deficiency of yang of the spleen and kidney
B: accumulation of cold
C: consumption of body fluids
D: damp-heat in the large intestine
E: retention of food

37. Watery stool with undigested food implies ( ).
38. Blood in the stool with mucus and a burning sensation in the anus results from ( ).

A: a bitter taste in the mouth
B: a sweet and sticky sensation in the mouth
C: tastelessness
D: a salty taste in the mouth

39. Damp-heat in the spleen and stomach results in ( ).

40. The fire of the liver and gallbladder results in ( ).

A: excessive heat in the blood
B: failure of Qi to control the blood
C: stagnation of blood
D: disharmony of the Chong and Ren channels due to the obstruction of liver Qi
E: damp-heat in the Chong and Ren channels

41. A prolonged menstrual cycle with scanty, purplish-dark discharge or blood clots suggests ( ).
42. Menses of a shortened cycle, excessive menstrual flow, thick and deep red in colour relates mainly to ( ).
43. A profuse, thin, and light-coloured mentrual flow indicates ( ).

A: superficial and rolling pulse (*fu* and *hua mai*)
B: surging and rapid pulse (*hong* and *shuo mai*)
C: deep and hesitant pulse (*chen* and *se mai*)
D: string-taut and rolling pulse (*xuan* and *hua mai*)
E: thready and rapid pulse (*xi* and *shuo mai*)

44. Excessive heat in the interior results in a ( ).
45. Stagnation of blood due to accumulation of cold results in a ( ).
46. Liver fire with phlegm results in a ( ).
47. Heat syndromes due to a deficiency of yin results in a ( ).

A: superficial and thready, and is felt by the fingers to be without strength
B: like a fine thready string but is very distinct and clear
C: tight and forceful like a stretched rope
D: smooth and flowing like pearls rolling on a dish
E: broad, large and forceful like roaring waves which come on powerfully and fade away.

48. A surging pulse (*hong mai*) feels ( ).
49. A tense pulse (*jin mai*) feels ( ).
50. A soft pulse (*ru mai*) feels ( ).

V. Differentiation of Syndromes

A: Excess syndromes of phlegm-heat in the lung
B: Excess phlegm-dampness in the lung
C: invasion of the lung by wind-cold

D: accumulation of cold-phlegm in the lung
E: invasion of the lung by wind-heat
F: accumulation of phlegm-heat in the lung
G: injury of the lung by pathogenic dryness
H: a long-standing yin deficiency of the lung

1. Thick sputum with foul smell suggests (   ).
2. Dilute, clear and odourless sputum suggests (   ).
3. Cough in a coarse voice usually suggests (   ).
4. Cough in a clear voice usually suggests (   ).
5. Coarse breathing accompanied by asthma and rattling sound of sputum suggests (   ).
6. Dry cough with little sputum suggests (   ).

A: sustained high-grade fever
B: a slight fever occurring at a definite time of the day
C: a feverish sensation conveyed to the body surface from the inteiror
D: a feverish sensation on the palms of the hands and soles of the feet

7. (   ) often indicates excess of heat in the interior due to invasion by exogenous pathogenic heat
8. (   ) often indicate(s) endogenous heat caused by deficiency of yin
9. (   ) often indicate(s) transmission of exogenous pathogens from the exterior to the interior.

A: weakness of the spleen and stomach
B: retention of food
C: hyperactivity of fire of the liver and gallbladder
D: damp-heat in the spleen

10. Stickiness and sweet taste in the mouth most likely suggests (   ).
11. A bitter taste in the mouth suggests (   ).
12. Foul belching and acid regurgitation suggests (   ).
13. Poor appetite, loose stools and fullness in the epigastrium and abdomen suggests (   ).

A: accumulation of damp-heat in the kidney and urinary bladder
B: deficiency-cold of the kidney and urinary bladder
C: deficiency of the spleen and kidney, accompanied by fluid retention

14. Scanty urine is most likely caused by (   ).
15. Frequent urination with clear urine suggests (   ).
16. Frequent urination scanty in amount and deep-yellow in colour suggests (   ).

A: deficiency syndrome
B: intestinal parasites
C: stagnation of Qi and blood
D: retention of food or phlegm
E: invasion of channels and collaterals by pathogenic wind
F: obstruction of channels and collaterals by cold-dampness
17. Fixed pain is often due to ( ).
18. Pain which is alleviated by pressure suggests ( ).
19. Pain which is aggravated by pressure suggests ( ).
20. Migrating pain is often due to ( ).

A: heat syndrome of the excess type
B: cold syndrome of the deficiency type
C: stagnation of Qi and blood
D: deficiency of blood
21. Post-menstrual lower abdominal pain which is reduced by pressing and accompanied by a scanty reddish menstrual flow suggests ( ).
22. Excess menstrual flow which is a deep-red colour and of a shortened cycle suggests ( ).
23. A prolonged menstrual cycle with a scanty light-coloured discharge suggests ( ).
24. Pre-menstrual distending pain in the lower abdomen which is aggravated by pressure, and a dark purplish menstrual flow with clots suggests ( ).

A: flare-up of liver fire
B: deficiency of the blood in the liver
C: stagnation of cold in the liver channel
D: depression of liver Qi
25. Hypochondriac and lower abdominal distention and pain, and a distending sensation in the breasts suggests ( ).
26. Dizziness and distending sensation in the head suggests ( ).
27. Dizziness and numbness of the limbs suggests ( ).

A: retention of food in the stomach
B: retention of fluid in the stomach due to cold
C: hyperactivity of fire of the stomach
28. Pain in the epigastric region which is aggravated by cold and alleviated by warmth suggests ( ).
29. Pain in the epigastric region accompanied by foul belching suggests ( ).

30. Burning pain in the epigastrium accompanied by preference for cold dirnks suggests ( ).

A: dryness of the lung due to a deficiency of yin
B: deficiency of yang of the spleen
C: deficiency of kidney yang
D: invasion of exogenous pathogenic heat

31. Dry cough with scanty or no sputum, accompanied by afternoon fever, suggests ( ).
32. A cough with excessive sputum which becomes more severe in winter, and accompanied by anorexia suggests ( ).
33. Needling with the reinforcing method combined with moxibustion can be applied to the syndrome of ( ).
34. Acupuncture without moxibustion is best applied to ( ).

A: deficiency of spleen yang
B: deficiency of kidney yang
C: dampness and heat in the intestine
D: cold and dampness in the intestine

35. Watery diarrhea with abdominal pain and borborymus suggests ( ).
36. Loose stool with undigested food suggests ( ).
37. Slight abdominal pain, borborygmus and diarrhea once or several times each morning at dawn suggests ( ).
38. Diarrhea with yellow, hot, loose and fetid stools suggests ( ).

A: Excessive anger
B: Excessive grief, melancholy and meditation
C: Excessive joy or fear and fright

39. ( ) may cause mental restlessness and give rise to palpitation, insomnia, irritability, anxiety and even mental disorders.
40. ( ) may cause dysfunction of the liver and its ability to promote unrestraint and patency of vital energy. This in turn will give rise to pain and distention in the costal and hypochondriac region, mental depression and irascibility.
41. ( ) may cause dysfunction of the spleen and stomach in its function of transportation and transformation, and cause anorexia and abdominal fullness and distention after meals.

A: existence of heat
B: existence of cold or deficiency of blood

C: stagnation of blood or severe pain

42. A patient with a red complexion suggests ( ).
43. A patient with a bluish-purple complexion suggests ( ).
44. A patient with a pale complexion suggests ( ).

A: retention of food
B: invasion by the exogenous cold-damp
C: retention of phlegm and dampness in the interior
D: invasion by the pestilential pathogens

45. A white, sticky tongue coating usually suggests ( ).
46. A thick, white tongue coating usually suggests ( ).
47. A dry, white coating usually suggests ( ).

A: A thin, yellow tongue coating
B: A thick, yellow tongue coating
C: A yellow, sticky tongue coating
D: A dry, yellow tongue coating

48. ( ) usually suggests persistent accumulation of the food in the stomach and intestine.
49. ( ) usually suggests invasion of the lung by wind-heat.
( ) usually suggests accumulation of heat in the stomach and intestine which results in damage to yin.
50. ( ) usually suggests accumulation of damp-heat in the interior or blockage of the lungs by phlegm-heat.

A: diarrhea with undigested food in the stool and clear urine in increased volume
B: nasal obstruction, soreness or itching of the throat
C: rough and chapped skin and dryness of the throat
D: heaviness and a sensation of distention in the head as though it were tightly bandaged, and a sticky and sweetish taste in the mouth
E: carbuncle, furuncle and ulcer with local heat and redness, swelling, and pain

51. The symptom(s) indicating being affected by pathogenic wind include(s) ( ).
52. The symptom(s) indicating being affected by pathogenic cold include(s) ( ).
53. The symptom(s) indicating being affected by pathogenic dampness include(s) ( ).
54. The symptom(s) indicating being affected by pathogenic dryness include(s) ( ).
55. The symptom(s) indicating being affected by pathogenic fire include(s) ( ).

VI. Techniques of Acupuncture, Moxibustion and Cupping

A: the point Neiguan (P 6)
B: the point Huantiao (G 30)
C: the point Dicang (St 4)
D: the point Guanyuan (Ren 4)

1. Insertion of the needle by pinching up the skin applies to ( ).
2. Insertion of the needle with the help of the puncturing and pressing hands applies to ( ).
3. Inserting the needle with the fingers strethching the skin applies to ( ).

A: Neiguan (P 6)
B: Huantiao (GB 30)

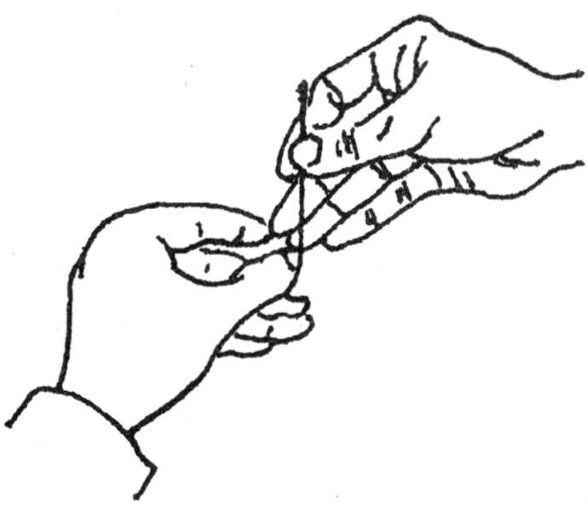

Fig. 3

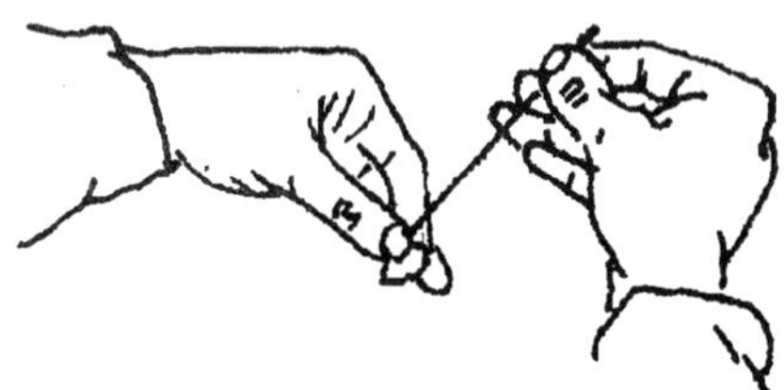

Fig. 4

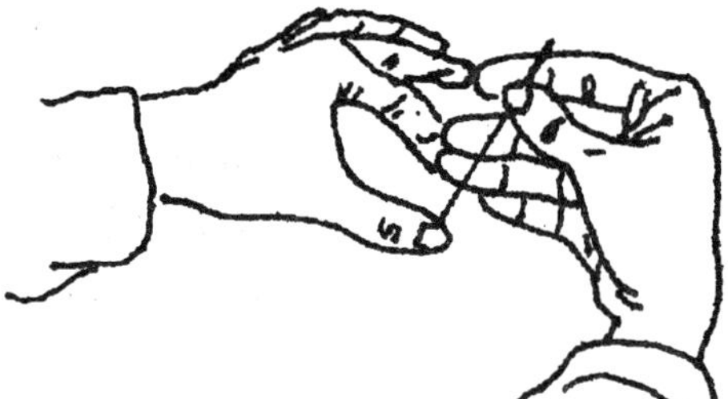

Fig. 5

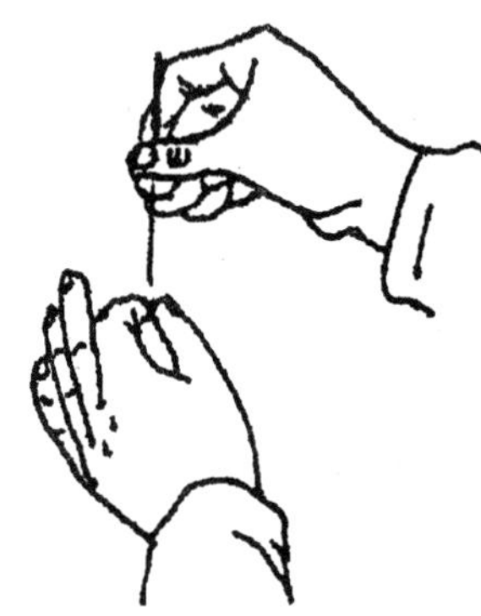

Fig. 6

C: Guanyuan (Ren 4)
D: Zanzhu (UB 2)
4. In Fig. 3, the point which the needle is inserted would be ( ).
5. In Fig. 4, the point which the needle is inserted would be ( ).
6. In Fig. 5, the point which the needle is inserted would be ( ).
7. In Fig. 6, the point which the needle is inserted would be ( ).

VII. Treatment of Diseases

A. Pishu (UB 20), Shenshu (UB 23), Qihai (Ren 6), Zusanli (St 36)
B: Zhongji (Ren 3), Hegu (LI 4), Xuehai (Sp 10), Xingjian (Liv 2)
C: Zhongji (Ren 3), Ciliao (UB 32), Diji (Sp 8)
D: Mingmen (Du 4), Shenshu (UB 23), Guanyuan (Ren 4), Zusanli (St 36), Dahe (K 1 2)
E: Daimai (GB 26), Baihuanshu (UB 30), Qihai (Ren 6), Sanyinjiao (Sp 6)
1. The prescription used to treat amenorrhea caused by blood deficiency is ( ).
2. The prescription used to treat dysmenorrhea caused by excess syndrome is ( ).

A: Shenmen (H 7), Sanyinjiao (Sp 6), Xinshu (UB 15), Pishu (UB 20), Jueyinshu (UB 14)
B: Shenmen (H 7), Sanyinjiao (Sp 6), Xinshu (UB 15), Shenshu (UB 23), Taixi (K 3)
C: Shenmen (H 7), Sanyinjiao (Sp 6), Weishu (UB 21), Zusanli (St 36)
D: Shenmen (H 7), Sanyinjiao (Sp 6), Xinshu (UB 15), Danshu (UB 19), Daling (P 7)
E: Shenmen (H 7), Sanyinjiao (Sp 6), Ganshu (UB 18), Jianshi (P 5), Taichong (Liv 3)
3. The prescription which is the best selection to treat insomnia caused by deficiency of both the heart and spleen would be ( ).
4. The prescription which is the best in treating insomnia caused by disharmony of the spleen and stomach Would be ( ).

A: Xinshu (UB 15), Ganshu (UB 18), Pishu (BU 20), Shenmen (H 7), Fenglong (St 40)
B: Dazhui (DU 14), Fengfu (Du 16), Shuigou (Du 26), Neiguan (P 6), Fenglong (St 40)
C: Jiuwei (Ren 15), Dazhui (Du 14), Yaoqi (Extra 19), Jianshi (P 5), Fenglong

(St 41)

D: Fengchi (GB 20), Ganshu (UB 18), Shenshu (UB 23), Xingjian (Liv 2), Fenglong (St 40)

E: Zhongwan (Ren 12), Neiguan (P 6), Pishu (UB 20), Jiexi (St 41), Fenglong (St 40)

5. The prescription commonly used in treating epilepsy is ( ).

6. The prescription commonly used in treating mania with emotional excitement is ( ).

7. The prescription used in treating insanity with emotional depression is ( ).

A: Baihui (Du 20), Tongtian (UB 7), Ahshi point(s), Xingjian (Liv 2)

B: Shangxing (DU 23), Touwei (St 8), Ahshi point(s), Hegu (LI 4)

C: Houding (Du 19), Dazhui (Du 14), Ahshi point(s), Kunlun (UB 60)

D: Fengchi (GB 20), Baihui (Du 20), Xuanlu (GB 5), Xiaxi (GB 43), Xingjian (Liv 2)

E: Baihui (Du 20), Qihai (Ren 6), Ganshu (UB 18), Pishu (UB 20), Shenshu (UB 23) , Zusanli (St 36)

8. The prescription used in treating parietal headache caused by the invasion of exogenous wind into channels and collaterals is ( ).

9. The prescription used in treating headache caused by a flare-up of liver yang is ( ).

A: Zhongwan (Ren 12), Qimen (Liv 14), Neiguan (P 6), Zusanli (St 36), Yanglingquan (GB 34)

B: Zhongwan (Ren 12), Zhangmen (Liv 13), Neiguan (P 6), Zusanli (St 36), Pishu (UB 20), Weishu (UB 21)

C: Zhongwan (Ren 12), Shenque (Ren 8), Guanyuan (Ren 4), Zusanli (St 36), Gongsun (Sp 4)

D: Zhongwan (Ren 12), Qihai (Ren 6), Zhangmen (Liv 3), Zusanli (St 36), Pishu (U B 20), Weishu (UB 21)

E: Zhongwan (Ren 12), Qihai (Ren 6), Tianshu (St 25), Zusanli (St 36), Neiting (St 44)

10. The prescription used in treating stomache caused by a deficiency of the spleen and stomach is ( ).

11. The prescripiton used in treating abdominal pain caused by a deficiency of spleen yang is ( ).

12. The prescription used in treating abdominal pain caused by the accumulation of exogenous cold is ( ).

A: the Back-Shu points

B: the Front-Mu points
C: the eight confluent points
D: the Ying-Spring points
E: the Luo-Connecting points

13. The points effective in treating febrile diseases are ( ).

14. According to *Classic on Medical Problems*, the points which are the best selection to treat diseases of the Fu organs are ( ).

15. According to *Classic on Medical Problems*, the points punctured as the best selected to treat diseases of the Zang organs are ( ).

16. The points selected for acupuncture to treat disorders of the two externally-internally related channels are ( ).

A: Chengshan (B 57)
B: Baihui (Du 20)
C: Erbai (Extra 31)
D: Changqiang (Du 1)
E: Laogong (P 8)

17. By using the theory "selecting the point along the channel" the point which is the best selection to treat hemorrhoids is ( ).

18. By using the theory of divergent channels, the point which is the best selection to treat hemorrhoids is ( ).

19. By using clinical experience without channel and collateral theory the point which is the best selection for treating hemorrhoids is ( ).

A: Hegu (LI 4), Jiache (St 6), Neiting (St 44), Waiguan (SJ 5), Fengchi (GB 20)
B: Hegu (LI 4), Jiache (St 6), Xiaguan (S 7), Taixi (K 3), Xingjian (Liv 2)
C: Hegu (LI 4), Shaoshang (Lu 11), Chize (Lu 5), Guanchong (SJ 1), Xiangu (St 43)
D: Taixi (K 3), Zhaohai (K 6), Yuji (Lu 10)
E: Hegu (LI 4), Lieque (Lu 7), Yingxiang (LI 20), Bitong (Extra 10), Yintang (Extra 2)

20. The prescription recommended for patients suffering from rhinorrhea is ( ).

21. The prescription commonly used in treating toothache caused by invasion of wind fire is ( ).

22. The prescription which is the best selection to relieve toothache caused by a deficiency of yin is ( ).

23. The prescription selected to treat sore throat caused by excessive heat is ( ).

A: as a local point
B: as a distal point
C: according to the principle of selecting upper points for the disorders of lower areas
D: basing on the experience that this point is an effective one in treating traumatic lower back pain and rigidity (In the prescription for treatment of lower back pain)

24. Bloodletting at Weizhong (UB 40) is selected ( ).
25. Feiyang (UB 58) is selected ( ).
26. Yaoyangguan (Du 3) is selected ( ).
27. Shuigou (Du 26) is selected ( ).

A: selection of local points
B: selection of remote points
C: selection of points along the channel governing the diseased areas
D: selection of points along channels associated with the diseased channels
E: selection of multiple points along several channels

28. Weizhong (UB 40) for lower back pain is according to ( ).
29. Yaoyangguan (Du 3) and Dachangshu (UB 25) for lower back pain are according to ( ).
30. In case of muscular rheumatism of the lower limbs with marked symptoms on the anterior lateral aspect, Biguan (St 31), Liangqiu (St 34), Zusanli (St 36), Fengshi (GB 31) and Yanglingquan (GB 34) are the best choice according to ( ).
31. In case of palpitation (caused by involvement of heart channel) the point Fuliu (K 7) can be employed according to ( ).

A: asthma caused by a deficiency of the lung
B: asthma caused by a deficiency of the kidney
C: asthma caused by wind-cold

32. Short and rapid breathing, weak and low voice and hidrosis usually suggests ( ).
33. The points Feishu (UB 13), Taiyuan (LU 9) and Zusanli (St 36) can be prescribed in treating ( ).
34. The points Shenshu (UB 23), Mingmen (Du 4), Qihai (Ren 6) and Tanzhong (Ren 17) can be prescribed in treating ( ).
35. Asthma, dyspnea upon exertion, and eversion to cold with cold extremities can be diagnosed as ( ).

A: Lieque (Lu 7), Hegu (LI 4), Feishu (UB 13), Chize (LU 5)
B: Pishu (UB 20), Zhongwan (Ren 12), Zusanli (St 36), Feishu (UB 13),

Gaohuangshu (UB 43), Fenglong (St 40)
C: Feishu (UB 13), Zhongfu (Lu 1), Lieque (Lu 7), Zhaohai (K 6)
36. The prescription used in treating cough by exogenous pathogens is ( ).
37. The prescription used in treating cough caused by dryness of the lung due to deficiency of yin is ( ).
38. The prescription used in treating cough caused by deficiency of spleen yang is ( ).

A: to treat weakness of the spleen
B: to treat borborygmus, vomiting and diarrhea
C: to treat cough and asthma
D: to treat vomiting blood, wasting and consumptive diseases
E: to treat muscular atrophy and weakness of the joints
F: to treat a Qi deficiency with a weak pulse
G: to treat painful joints and rheumatism
H: to treat apoplexy and paralysis
39. The influential point of the Fu organs, Zhongwan (Ren 12), can be used ( ).
40. The influential point of the blood, Geshu (UB 17), can be used ( ).
41. The influential point of the marrow, Xuanzhong (GB 39), can be used ( ).
42. The influential point of the bones, Dashu (UB 11), can be used ( ).
43. The influential point of the Zang organs, Zhangmen (Liv 13), can be used ( ).
44. The influential point of the Qi, Tanzhong (Ren 17), can be used ( ).
45. The influential point of the tendon and muscle, Yanglingquan (GB 34), can be used ( ).
46. The influential point of the vessels, Taiyuan (Lu 9), can be used ( ).

The Xi-Cleft points have the functions of treating acute diseases occurring in their respective organs.

A: menstrual pain
B: hemoptysis
C: epigastric pain
D: borborygmus and abdominal pain
47. Kongzui (Lu 6) is effective in ( ).
48. Wenliu (LI 7) is effective for ( ).
49. Liangqiu (St 34) is used to treat ( ).
50. Diji (Sp 8) is often prescribed for ( ).

Solutions to the Exercises

I.

1. D; 2. E; 3. B; 4. B; 5. B; 6. D; 7. C; 8. A; 9. B; 10. A.

II.

1. B, F, G; 2. A; 3. C, I, M; 4. E, H, L; 5. K, J, D; 6. C; 7. B; 8. C; 9. D; 10 . A; 11. B; 12. B; 13. E; 14. D; 15. A; 16. C; 17. C; 18. E; 19. F; 20. A; 21. B ; 22. D; 23. D; 24. B; 25. C; 26. A; 27. B; 28. A; 29. A; 30. B; 31. A.

III.

1. D; 2. E; 3. C; 4. B; 5. E; 6. B; 7. C; 8. E; 9. A; 10. C; 11. A; 12. D; 13. B ; 14. E; 15. C; 16. B; 17. A; 18. D; 19. E; 20. E; 21. B; 22. A; 23. C; 24. D; 2 5. C; 26. A; 27. B; 28. C; 29. D; 30. B, D; 31. E, A; 32. C.

IV.

1. A; 2. E; 3. D; 4. E; 5. A; 6. C; 7. A; 8. D; 9. B; 10. D; 11. C; 12. A; 13. E; 14. D; 15. A; 16. B; 17. D; 18. C; 19. A; 20. C; 21. E; 22. B; 23. D; 24. E; 2 5. A; 26. B; 27. A; 28. B; 29. E; 30. C; 31. E; 32. D; 33. E; 34. B; 35. C; 36. A; 37. A; 38. D; 39. B; 40. A; 41. C; 42. A; 43. B; 44. B; 45. C; 46. D; 47. E; 48. E; 49. C; 50. A.

V.

1. F, A; 2. D; 3. C, D; 4. E, F; 5. A, B, F; 6. G, H; 7. A; 8. B, C, D; 9. A; 10. D; 11. C; 12. B; 13. A; 14. C; 15. B; 16. A; 17. C; 18. A; 19. B, C, D; 20. E; 21. D; 22. A; 23. B; 24. C; 25. D; 26. A; 27. B; 28. B; 29. A; 30. C; 31. A; 32. B ; 33. B, C; 34. A, D; 35. D; 36. A; 37. B; 38. C; 39. C; 40. A; 41. B; 42. A; 43. C; 44. B; 45. B, C; 46. A; 47. D; 48. B; 49. A, D; 50. C; 51. B; 52. A; 53. D; 54. C; 55. E.

VI.

1. C; 2. B; 3. D; 4. A; 5. B; 6. C; 7. D.

VII.

1. A; 2. C; 3. A; 4. C; 5. C; 6. B; 7. A; 8. A; 9. D; 10. B; 11. D; 12. C; 13. D ; 14. B; 15. A; 16. E; 17. B; 18. A; 19. C; 20. E; 21. A; 22. B; 23. C; 24. D; 25. B; 26. A; 27. C; 28. B, C; 29. A; 30. E; 31. D; 32. A; 33. A; 34. B; 35. B; 36. A; 37. C; 38. B; 39. B; 40. D; 41. H; 42. E; 43. A; 44. C; 45. E; 46. F; 47. B; 48. D; 49. C; 50. A.

"C" Type Questions

These contain four options (lettered A to D) that are followed by one or two questions. For EACH question select the answer that you consider to be correct. Each option may be selected more than once or not at all.

Example:

For each numbered statement select the answer most closely associated with it.

A: Ahshi points are the main points used

B: Local and distal points of the involved channels may be used

C: Both A and B may be used

D: Neither A nor B may be used

in treatment of acute sprain ( ).

The correct answer is C and would be marked in ( ).

I. Yin-Yang and the Five Elements

A: Shu-Stream points

B: He-Sea points

C: both A and B

D: neither A nor B

1. The attribution of ( ) in the five-Shu points to the Five Elements is earth.
2. The attribution of ( ) in the five-Shu points to the Five Elements is water.
3. The attribution of ( ) in the five-Shu points to the Five Elements is metal.

A: definite

B: relative

C: both A and B

D: neither A nor B

1. The attribution of ( ) in the five-Shu points to the Five Elements is earth.
2. The attribution of ( ) in the five-Shu points to the Five Elements is water.
3. The attribution of ( ) in the five-Shu points to the Five Elements is metal.

A: definite

B: relative

C: both A and B

D: neither A nor B

4. The yin-yang nature of things is ( ).
5. the five categories of Zang-Fu organs classified according to the Five Elements are ( ).

A: reinforce the "mother" for Xu syndrome

B: reduce the "son" for Shi syndrome
C: both A and B
D:neither A nor B
6. The basic principle of treatment according to the relationship of overacting is ( ).
7. The basic principle for treating deficiency of kidney yin and hyperactivity of heart fire includes ( ).

II. Zang-Fu, Qi, Blood and Body Fluid

A: the liver maintaining patency for the flow of Qi
B: the kidney stores the essence
C: both A and B
D: neither A nor B
1. The function(s) related to reproduction include(s) ( ).
2. The function(s) related to movements of the extremities include(s) ( ).
3. The function(s) related to emotional activities include(s) ( ).

A: The control of respiration
B: the control of water metabolism
C: both A and B
D: neither A nor B
4. The relationship between the heart and liver exists in ( ).
5. The relationship between the lung and kidney exists in ( ).

A: polyuria
B: oliguria
C: both A and B
D: neither A nor B
6. A deficiency of kidney yin results in ( ).
7. A deficiency of spleen yang results in ( ).
8. A deficiency of kidney yang results in ( ).

A: constipation
B: diarrhea
C: both A and B
D: neither A nor B
9. A deficiency of yang can be the cause of ( ).
10. A deficiency of yin can be the cause of ( ).

11. A deficiency of Qi can be the cause of (   ).

III. The Channels, Collaterals and Acupoints

A: the channel of Foot-Yangming
B: the channel of Hand-Yangming
C: both A and B
D: neither A nor B

1. The channel that distributes to the upper teeth is (   ).
2. The channel that distributes to the lower teeth is (   ).

A: Hegu (LI 4)
B: Zhiyin (UB 67)
C: both A and B
D: neither A nor B

3. The point(s) usually selected for moxibustion to correct the position of fetus is/are (   ).
4. The point(s) to which acupuncture can not be applied during pregnancy is/are (   ).

A: Pishu (UB 20), Zhangmen (Liv 13)
B: Dachangshu (UB 25), Tianshu (St 25)
C: both A and B
D: neither A nor B

5. The points often selected for treating chronic diarrhea are (   ).
6. The points often selected to treat habitual constipation are (   ).

A: a Luo-Connecting point
B: one of the eight confluent points
C: both A and B
D: neither A nor B

7. The point Neiguan (P 6) is (   ).
8. The point Waiguan (SJ 5) is (   ).
9. The point Shangguan (GB 3) is (   ).
10. The point Xiaguan (St 7) is (   ).

IV. Diagnostic Methods

A: failure of the blood to nourish the heart due to deficiency of both the

heart and spleen
B: hyperactivity of heart fire
C: both A and B
D: neither A nor B
1. Insomnia accompanied by mental restlessness and dream-disturbed sleep usually indicates (   ).

A: menses of a shortened cycle
B: deep red menses which are excessive in amount
C: both A and B
D: neither A nor B
2. Dysmenorrhea caused by excessive heat is suggested by (   ).
3. Dysmenorrhea caused by heat due to deficiency of yin is suggested by (   ).

A: distending pain in the costal and hypochondriac regions, and fullness in the chest
B: fixed stabbing pain in the hypochondriac region, or pain intensified when pressure is applied and at night
C: both A and B
D: neither A nor B
4. Stagnation of blood is usually manifested in (   ).
5. Stagnation of qi is usually manifested in (   ).

V. Differentiaiton of Syndromes

A: invasion by wind-heat
B: invaison by wind-cold
C: both A and B
D: neither A nor B
1. In exterior syndrome, sweating suggests (   ).

A: deficiency of yang Qi
B: weakness of defensive Qi
C: both A and B
D: neither A nor B
2. The causative factor(s) of frequent spontaneous sweating exacerbated by slight exertion is/are (   ).

A: accumulation of phlegm-damp in the interior

B: deficiency of Qi and blood
C: both A and B
D: neither A nor B

3. Lethargy accompanied by dizziness and heaviness of the head usually suggests ( ).

A: weakness and cold of the spleen and stomach
B: deficiency of spleen kidney yang
C: both A and B
D: neither A nor B

4. Constant diarrhea before daybreak usually relates to ( ).

A: palpitation, dream-disturbed sleep, vertigo and poor memory
B: poor appetite, abdominal distention, loose stool, and lassitude
C: both A and B
D: neither A nor B

5. Deficiency of blood of the heart and liver is manifested in ( ).
6. Deficiency of Qi of the spleen is manifested in ( ).
7. Deficiency of the heart and spleen is manifested in ( ).

A: vertigo and tinnitus
B: afternoon fever and night sweating
C: both A and B
D: neither A nor B

8. Damp-heat of the liver and gallbladder is often manifested in ( ).
9. Deficiency of liver yin is often manifested in ( ).

A: deficiency of liver yin
B: flare-up of liver yang
C: both A and B
D: neither A nor B

10. Wiry (string-taut) pulse (*xuan mai*) often suggests ( ).
11. Thready pulse (*xi mai*) often suggests ( ).

A: deficiency syndrome
B: cold syndrome
C: both A and B
D: neither A nor B

12. A prolonged menstrual cycle with scanty light-coloured discharge usually suggests ( ).
13. Pre-menstrual distending pain in the lower abdominal region which intensi-

fies when pressure is applied, and a dark purplish menstrual flow with clots suggests ( ).

14. Post-menstrual lower abdominal pain that is reduced when pressure is applied and a light-reddish menstrual flow scanty in amount suggests ( ).

VI. Techniques of Acupuncture, Moxibusiton and Cupping

A. three-edged needles
B: subcutaneous needles
C: both A and B
D: neither A nor B

1. ( ) is indicated in treating headache and/or hypertension.
2. ( ) is indicated in treating acute lumbar sprain, tonsillitis, etc.

A: The deeper a needle is inserted, the better the result.
B: The needle is inserted only deep enough to produce the arrival of Qi (De Qi).
C: both A and B
D: neither A nor B

3. Which of the above statements regarding the depth of needle insertion is correct? ( )

A: the same patient during one treatment
B: the same patient over several treatments
C: both A and B
D: neither A nor B

4. Both reinforcement and reduction needling techniques can be applied to ( ).

A: The needle is too long
B: The inserting technique is inappropriate
C: both A and B
D: neither A nor B

5. Refer to Fig. 7 Which of the statement would you consider tobe true? ( )

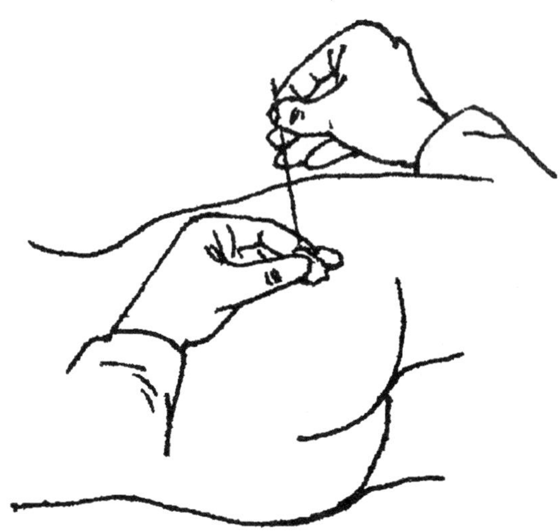

Fig. 7

VII. Treatment of Diseases

A: Hegu (LI 4)
B: Neiting (St 44)
C: both A and B
D: neither A nor B

1. In treating a toothache of the upper teeth, the point(s) selected would be ( ).
2. In treating a toothache of the lower teeth, the point(s) selected would be ( ).

A: Shuigou (Du 26), Dazhui (Du 14), Hegu (LI 4), Shixuan (Extra 30), Yanglingquan (GB 34), Taichong (Liv 3)
B: Zhongwan (Ren 12), Zhangmen (Liv 13), Qihai (Ren 6), Tianshu (St 25), Zusanli (St 36), Xingjian (Liv 2)
C: both A and B
D: neither A nor B

3. The prescription(s) commonly used in the treatment of acute infantile convulsion would be ( ).
4. The prescription(s) commonly used in the treatment of chronic infantile convulsion would be ( ).

A: Qimen (Liv 14), Zhigou (SJ 6), Yanglingquan (GB 34), Zusanli (St 36), Taichong (GB 9)
B: Qimen (Liv 14), Sanyinjiao (Sp 6), Ganshu (UB 18), Shenshu (UB 23), Zusanli (St 36)
C: both A and B
D: neither A nor B

5. The prescription(s) indicated in hypochondriac pain of an excessive syndrome is/are ( ).
6. The prescription(s) indicated in hypochondriac pain of a deficient syndrome is/are ( ).

A: mental disturbance
B: febrile diseases
C: both A and B
D: neither A nor B

7. Some points on the Ren channel are indicated in ( ).
8. Some points on the Du channel are indicated in ( ).

A: Shenshu (UB 23), Mingmen (Du 4), Sanyinjiao (Sp 6), Guanyuan (Ren 4)
B: Guanyuan (Ren 4), Zhongji (Ren 3), Sanyinjiao (Sp 6), Shenshu (UB 23),

Pangguangshu (UB 28)
C: both A and B
D: neither A nor B
9. The prescription(s) applicable in treating impotence is/are ( ).
10. The prescription(s) applicable in treating nocturnal emission is/are ( ).
11. The prescription(s) applicable in treating enuresis is/are ( ).

A: Points on the liver channel
B: Points on the gallbladder channel
C: both A and B
D: neither A nor B
12. For the treatment of hypochondriac pain, ( ) should be punctured.

A: the Front-Mu point of the urinary bladder
B: the Back-Shu and Front-Mu points of the kidney and the Back-Shu point of the urinary bladder.
C: both A and B
D: neither A nor B
13. In treating nocturnal enuresis ( ) is/are the main point(s) for tonification of the kidney Qi.
14. In treating retention of urine ( ) should be chosen as the main point(s) (in accordance with the principle of treating acute symptoms).

A: Hegu (LI 4) is selected
B: Lieque (Lu 7) is selected
C: both A and B
D: neither A nor B
15. in treating disease caused by exogenous factors ( ).
16. in treating stiff neck and headache ( ).
17. in treating facial paralysis ( ).
18. in treating sore throat ( ).
19. in treating hyperhydrosis or anhydrosis ( ).

A: Using Back-Shu points and points on the liver channel as main points is suitable for
B: Using filiform needles with even movements is suitable for
C: both A and B are suitable for
D: neither A nor B is suitable for
20. the treatment of hypochondriac pain due to excess syndrome ( ).
21. the treatment of hypochondriac pain due to deficiency syndrome ( ).

A: Xinshu (UB 15), Shenshu (UB 23), Taixi (K 3)
B: Pishu (UB 20), Xingshu (UB 15), Yinbai (Sp 1)
C: both A and B
D: neither A nor B

22. The prescription used in treating insomnia caused by an upward disturbance of liver fire would be ( ).
23. The prescription used in treating somnia caused by a deficiency of the spleen and blood would be ( ).
24. The prescription used in treating insomnia caused by a dysfunction of the stomach would be ( ).
25. The prescription used in treating somnia cuased by the disharmony of the heart and kidney would be ( ).

A: the channel of Hand-Yangming
B: the channel of Foot-Yangming
C: both A and B
D: neither A nor B

26. In treating a toothache due to the invasion by wind-heat, the points employed are mainly on ( ).
27. In treating a toothache due to a deficiency of the kidney, the points selected are mainly on ( ).
28. In treating a toothache due to an excess syndrome, the points used are mainly on ( ).

Solutions to the Exercises

I.
1. C; 2. B; 3. D; 4. B; 5. A; 6. D; 7. D.

II.
1. C; 2. D; 3. A; 4. D; 5. C; 6. B; 7. B; 8. C; 9. C; 10. A; 11. C.

III.
1. A; 2. B; 3. B; 4. C; 5. C; 6. B; 7. C; 8. C; 9. D; 10. D.

IV.
1. B; 2. C; 3. D; 4. B; 5. A.

V.
1. A; 2. B; 3. A; 4. B; 5. A; 6. B; 7. C; 8. D; 9. C; 10. C; 11. D; 12. C; 13 . D; 14. A.

VI.
1. C; 2. A; 3. B; 4. C; 5. D.

VII.

1. B; 2. A; 3. A; 4. B; 5. A; 6. B; 7. A; 8. C; 9. A; 10. B; 11. B; 12. C; 13. C; 14. A; 15. C; 16. B; 17. C; 18. C; 19. A; 20. D; 21. C; 22. D; 23. A; 24. D; 2 5. C; 26. C; 27. B; 28. C.

"K" Type Questions

These have a stem and four options, ONE OR MORE OF WHICH MAY BE CORRECT. These questions are answered by using the following keys.
Only 1,2,3 correct......Fill in ( ) with A
Only 1 and 3 correct......Fill in ( ) with B
Only 2 and 4 correct......Fill in ( ) with C
Only 4 correct......Fill in ( ) with D
All answers are correct......Fill in ( ) with E

Directions Summarized
A: 1,2,3
B: 1,3
C: 2,4
D: 4
E: all answers are correct

Example:
Which of the following symptoms indicate(s) an exterior cold syndrome? ( )
(1) Chills
(2) Fever
(3) No sweating
(4) Loose stools
1, 2, 3 are correct, thus A is the correct answer.

I. Yin-Yang and the Five Elements

1. Which of the following properties belong to yang? ( )
(1) moving
(2) nourishing
(3) warming

(4) moistening

2. Which of the following properties belong to yang? (　)

(1) brightness
(2) upward direction
(3) excitement
(4) inward direction

3. Which of the following properties belong to yin? (　)

(1) coldness
(2) inhibition
(3) stillness
(4) outward direction

4. Which of the following body parts belong to yang? (　)

(1) medial aspects of the four limbs
(2) the head
(3) the abdomen
(4) the back

5. Which of the following body parts belong to yin? (　)

(1) the abdomen
(2) the medial aspects of the four limbs
(3) the lower part
(4) the head

6. The basic theories of yin and yang include the theories of (　).

(1) the opposition
(2) the interdependence
(3) the inter-consuming-supporting relationship
(4) the inter-transforming relationship

7. According to the theory of the Five Elements, which of the following pertain to wood? (　)

(1) sour
(2) wind
(3) east
(4) tongue

8. According to the theory of the Five Elements, which of the following pertain to fire? (　)

(1) red
(2) east

(3) joy
(4) dryness

9. According to the theory of the Five Elements, which of the following pertain to wood? (　)

(1) bitter
(2) anger
(3) hair
(4) the gallbladder

10. According to the theory of the Five Elements, which of the following pertain to earth? (　)

(1) middle
(2) yellow
(3) the spleen
(4) the mouth

11. According to the theory of the Five Elements, which of the following pertain to metal? (　)

(1) pungent
(2) white
(3) autumn
(4) the small intestine

12. According to the theory of the Five Elements, which of the following pertain to water? (　)

(1) salty
(2) black
(3) cold
(4) the kidney

13. Which of the following relations belong to interpromoting between different elements? (　)

(1) wood to fire
(2) fire to water
(3) earth to metal
(4) metal to wood

14. Which of the following relations belong to interacting between different elements? (　)

(1) water to wood
(2) fire to metal

(3) earth to water
(4) wood to metal

15. Which of the following have interpromoting relationships? ( )
(1) the kidney and heart
(2) the spleen and lung
(3) the liver and spleen
(4) the kidney and liver

16. Which of the following have interacting relationships? ( )
(1) the liver and spleen
(2) the spleen and lung
(3) the heart and lung
(4) the kidney and liver

17. According to the theory of the Five Elements, the clinical manifestations belong to the liver include ( ).
(1) easy to be angry
(2) bitter taste in the mouth
(3) wiry pulse
(4) pale

18. Which of the following problems are due to counteracting among the Five Elements? ( )
(1) stagnation of the liver qi which attacks the spleen
(2) transmission of heart fire to the small intestine
(3) failure of the kidney to support the liver
(4) attack of the lung by liver fire

19. According to the theory of the Five Elements, the points belonging to metal include ( ).
(1) Shaoshang (L 11)
(2) Shangyang (LI 1)
(3) Neiting (S 44)
(4) Lingdao (H 4)

20. According to the principle of "reinforcing the mother," which of the following methods can be selected? ( )
(1) reinforcing the kidney to reinforce the liver
(2) reinforcing the kidney and heart
(3) reinforcing the earth to strengthen metal
(4) moving liver qi to help the spleen

II. Zang-Fu, Qi, Blood and Body Fluid

1. The function(s) of the heart include(s) ( ).

(1) dominating the blood and vessels
(2) moving the Qi
(3) housing the mind
(4) storing the blood

2. "The heart dominates the blood and vessel" means that ( ).

(1) the heart dominates the blood of the whole body
(2) the heart dominates the vessels of the whole body
(3) the heart is the motive force for blood circulation
(4) the heart produces the blood

3. The function of the heart in housing the mind is linked with ( ).

(1) consciousness
(2) spirit
(3) sleep
(4) memory

4. The heart dominating the blood and vessels means that ( ).

(1) the heart controls the blood in the vessels
(2) the heart produces the blood to support the vessles
(3) the heart regulates the amount of the blood circulating within the vessels
(4) the heart is the motive force for blood circulation

5. The heart ( ).

(1) dominates the blood and vessels
(2) manifests on the face
(3) houses the mind
(4) opens to the tongue

6. The liver regulates ( ).

(1) water metabolism of the whole body
(2) the volume of blood circulating in the body
(3) yin and yang of the whole body
(4) movement of Qi of the whole body

7. The liver ( ).

(1) stores blood
(2) maintains the free flow of Qi
(3) controls the tendons

(4) opens to the eye

8. The function of the liver for maintaining the free flow of Qi links with ( ).

(1) emotional activity
(2) ascending and descending function of the stomach and spleen
(3) secretion of the bile
(4) keeping the blood circulating in the vessels

9. Dysfunction of the liver for maintaining the free flow of Qi may affect ( ).

(1) secretion and excretion of the bile
(2) digestion
(3) emotion
(4) circulation of blood

10. The function of the lung in dominating Qi means ( ).

(1) dominating the Qi of the respiration
(2) maintaining the free flow of Qi
(3) dominating the Qi of the whole body
(4) absorbing nutrient substance

11. The functions of the lung include ( ).

(1) dominating Qi
(2) controlling respiration
(3) dominating dispersing and descending
(4) regulating the water passage

12. The function of the lung in regulating the water passage means ( ).

(1) absorbing nutrient substances from water
(2) keeping unrestrained pathways for the circulation of water
(3) storing water
(4) regulating the excretion of water

13. The lung ( ).

(1) dominates the skin
(2) dominates the muscles
(3) opens to the nose
(4) dominates the four limbs

14. The pectoral Qi is formed from ( ).

(1) the kidney Qi
(2) the essential Qi of water and food
(3) the defensive Qi

(4) the clear Qi inhaled by the lung

15. The pectoral Qi ( ).

(1) accumulates in the chest
(2) ascends to the throat
(3) dominates respiration
(4) promotes the heart's function

16. The functions of the spleen inclucde ( ).

(1) governing transportation and transformation
(2) regulating water passage
(3) controlling blood
(4) storing essence

17. The function of the spleen in transporting and transforming refers to ( ).

(1) digestion of food and water
(2) absorption of nutrient substances
(3) transmission of nutrient substances
(4) storing of nutrient substances

18. The function of the spleen in controlling blood means the spleen has the function of ( ).

(1) promoting the circulation of blood
(2) storing the blood
(3) manufacturing blood
(4) keeping the blood circulating within the vessels

19. The spleen has the functions of ( ).

(1) digesting food
(2) absorbing essence
(3) producing Qi and blood
(4) transforming dampness

20. The spleen ( ).

(1) dominates the muscles
(2) dominates the four limbs
(3) opens to the mouth
(4) manifests on the lips

21. The kidney has the function of ( ).

(1) storing essence
(2) dominating development and reproduction

(3) dominating water metabolism
(4) storing blood

22. The kidney ( ).
(1) opens to the ear
(2) dominates the bone
(3) dominates the urethra and anus orifices
(4) manifests in the hair

23. The kidney essence has the functions of ( ).
(1) producing marrow
(2) nourishing the bone
(3) nourishing the hair
(4) producing the blood

24. The main functions of the stomach are ( ).
(1) receiving food
(2) absorbing essence from food
(3) decomposing food
(4) transmission of food essence

25. The main functions of the gallbladder are ( ).
(1) producing bile
(2) storing bile
(3) digesting food
(4) excreting bile to the intestines

26. The main functions of the small intestine are ( ).
(1) receiving the food from the stomach
(2) separating the clear from the turbid
(3) absorbing essential substances and some of the water from the food
(4) transmitting the residue of the food to the large intestine and water to the bladder

27. The main functions of the large intestine are ( ).
(1) receiving the waste materials sent from the small intestin
(2) absorbing the fluid content of waste materials
(3) forming the waste materials into faces to be excreted
(4) separating the clear from the turbid substances

28. The main functions of the bladder include ( ).
(1) dominating water metabolism
(2) temporary storage of urine

(3) regulating water passage
(4) discharging urine

29. The main functions of the Sanjiao are ( ).
(1) to govern various forms of Qi
(2) to serve as the passage for the flow of Qi
(3) to serve as the pathway for body fluid
(4) to dominate the blood and vessels

30. The functions of the middle-Jiao are ( ).
(1) to digest food
(2) absorb essential substances
(3) to evaporate body fluids
(4) to transform nutrient substances into blood

31. The extraordinary Fu organs include ( ).
(1) the uterus
(2) the brain
(3) the gallbladder
(4) the Sanjiao

32. Acquired Qi includes ( ).
(1) Zong Qi (pectoral Qi)
(2) Wei Qi (defensive Qi)
(3) Ying qi (nutrient Qi)
(4) Yuan Qi (primary Qi)

33. Congenital Qi includes ( ).
(1) Zong Qi (pectoral Qi)
(2) Wei Qi (defensive Qi)
(3) Ying Qi (nutrient Qi)
(4) Yuan Qi (primary Qi)

34. The primary functions of Ying Qi (nutrient Qi) are ( ).
(1) controlling respiration
(2) producing blood
(3) producing water metabolism
(4) circulating with the blood

35. The functions of Wei Qi (defensive Qi) are ( ).
(1) protecting the body surface

(2) controlling the opening and closing of the pores
(3) moistening the skin and hair
(4) warming the Zang-Fu organs

36. The functions of Qi include ( ).
(1) promoting
(2) warming
(3) defending
(4) checking

37. The circulation of blood in the vessels depends on the functions of ( ).
(1) the heart
(2) the liver
(3) the spleen
(4) the kidney

38. The blood is transformed from ( ).
(1) food essence
(2) Ying Qi (nutrient Qi)
(3) kidney essence
(4) Zong Qi (pectoral Qi)

39. The components of the blood include ( ).
(1) Ying Qi (nutrient Qi)
(2) body fluid
(3) kidney essence
(4) Wei Qi (defensive Qi)

40. The formation and distribution of body fluid are linked with the normal functions of ( ).
(1) the spleen and stomach
(2) the lung
(3) the kidney
(4) the small intestine

41. Clinically, the Zang organ(s) most likely effected by emotional factors is/are ( ).
(1) the heart
(2) the liver
(3) the spleen
(4) the kidney

42. TCM attributes the formation of a tumour (or enlargement of the internal organs in the abdomen) to ( ).

(1) Qi stagnancy
(2) blood deficiency
(3) phlegm-damp
(4) blood stasis

43. The cause(s) of the formation of soft, movable nodules include(s) ( ).

(1) Qi stagnancy
(2) cold-damp
(3) superficial blood stasis
(4) phlegm retaind subcutaneously

44. The Zang-Fu organs that are related to emotional activities include ( ).

(1) the heart
(2) the brain
(3) the liver
(4) the kidney

45. Which of the following organs or channels relate(s) to normal menstruation? ( )

(1) the kidney
(2) the liver
(3) the Chong channel
(4) the Ren channel

III. The Channels, Collaterals and Acupoints

1. The channels distributing to the back of the body include ( ).

(1) the bladder channel
(2) the kidney channel
(3) the Du channel
(4) the Chong channel

2. The channels passing through the medial aspect of the legs include ( ).

(1) the liver channel
(2) the spleen channel
(3) the kidney channel
(4) the gallbladder channel

3. The channels linked with the throat include ( ).

(1) the lung channel
(2) the liver channel
(3) the kidney channel
(4) the stomach channel

4. The channels distributing to the cheek include ( ).

(1) the stomach channel
(2) the small intestine channel
(3) the large intestine channel
(4) the bladder channel

5. The channels linked with the "eye system" include ( ).

(1) the spleen channel
(2) the heart channel
(3) the kidney channel
(4) the liver channel

6. Besides the kidney and bladder, the kidney channel is linked with ( ).

(1) the liver
(2) the heart
(3) the lung
(4) the spleen

7. The channels distributing to the chest and abdomen include ( ).

(1) the kidney channel
(2) the stomach channel
(3) the spleen channel
(4) the liver channel

8. The channels linked with teeth include ( ).

(1) the stomach channel
(2) the kidney channel
(3) the large intestine channel
(4) the lung channel

9. The liver channel passes through ( ).

(1) the external genitalia
(2) the lower abdomen
(3) the costal and hypochondriac region
(4) the posterior aspect of the malleolus

10. Besides the liver, the channel is linked with (   ).
(1) the gallbladder
(2) the lung
(3) the stomach
(4) the heart

11. The channel(s) enteirng the brain include(s) (   ).
(1) the Du channel
(2) the liver channel
(3) the bladder channel
(4) the gallbladder channel

12. The channel(s) distributing to the ear include(s) (   ).
(1) Hand-Shaoyang
(2) Hand-Taiyang
(3) Foot-Taiyang
(4) Foot-Yangming

13. The channel(s) distributing to the lips include(s) (   ).
(1) the large intestine channel
(2) the liver channel
(3) the stomach channel
(4) the Ren channel

14. The channels distributing to the forehead include (   ).
(1) the stomach channel
(2) the liver channel
(3) the bladder channel
(4) the large intestine channel

15. The channel(s) entering the lung include(s) (   ).
(1) the heart channel
(2) the spleen channel
(3) the kidney channel
(4) the pericardium channel

16. The channel(s) meeting at Zhongji (Ren 3) and Guanyuan (Ren 4) are (   ).
(1) the spleen
(2) the liver
(3) the kidney
(4) the stomach

17. The indications the points of the three yang channels of the foot have in common are ( ).

(1) mental illness
(2) disorders of the eyes
(3) febrile diseases
(4) disorders of the ears

18. The indications the points of the three yang channels of the hand have in common are ( ).

(1) disorders of the forehead, face, nose, mouth and teeth
(2) disorders of the temporal and hypochondriac regions
(3) disorders of the occipital and scapula regions and mental illness
(4) disorders of the eye and throat and febrile diseases

19. The indications the points of the three yin channels of the foot have in common are ( ).

(1) disorders of the eye and throat
(2) disorders of the external genitalia
(3) mental illness
(4) gynaecological diseases

20. The indications the points of three yin channels of the hand have in common are ( ).

(1) mental illness
(2) febrile diseases
(3) disorders of the ear
(4) disorders of the chest

21. The indications the points of the Ren and Du channels have in common are ( ).

(1) disorders of Zang-Fu organs
(2) mental illness
(3) gynaecological disorders
(4) febrile diseases

22. Tanzhong (Ren 17) is one of ( ).

(1) the eight influential points
(2) the eight confluent points
(3) the Front-Mu points
(4) the Back-Shu points

23. Hegu (LI 4) is ( ).

(1) a Luo-Connecting point
(2) a Xi-Cleft point
(3) a Jing-River point
(4) a Yuan-Primary point

24. Lieque (L 7) is ( ).

(1) a Xi-Cleft point
(2) a Luo-Connecting point
(3) a Jing-River point
(4) a confluent point

25. Taiyuan (L 9) is ( ).

(1) a Shu-Stream point
(2) a Yuan-Primary point
(3) an influential point
(4) a Luo-Connecting point

26. Which of the following point(s) should be punctured with the patient's mouth open? ( ).

(1) Ermen (SJ 21)
(2) Tinggong (SI 19)
(3) Tinghui (G 2)
(4) Jiache (S 6)

27. The indication(s) of Quchi (LI 11) include(s) ( ).

(1) sore throat
(2) motor impairment of the upper extremities
(3) scrofula
(4) abdominal pain, vomiting, diarrhea

28. The indication(s) of Yingxiang (LI 20) is (are) ( ).

(1) nasal obstruction
(2) deviation of the mouth
(3) itching and swelling of the face
(4) pain and itching of the eye

29. The indication(s) of Chengshan (B 57) is/are ( ).

(1) lower back pain
(2) spasm of the gastrocnemius
(3) hemorrhoids

(4) dysmenorrhea

30. When Jingming (B 1) is punctured, which of the following things must be done ? ( )

(1) ask the patient to close his eyes
(2) push the eyeball gently to the lateral side
(3) puncture slowly 0.3-0.7 inch perpendicularly along the orbital wall
(4) refrain from twisting, lifting or thrusting the needle

31. Which of the following points is/are located 7 cun above the malleolus? ( )

(1) Yangjiao (G 35)
(2) Waiqiu (G 36)
(3) Feiyang (B 58)
(4) Zhongdu (Liv 6)

32. Which of the following points is/are at the level with the umbilicus? ( )

(1) Tianshu (St 25)
(2) Daimai (G 26)
(3) Daheng (Sp 15)
(4) Gaoshu (K 16)

33. Which of the following points is/are at the level of the lower border of the spinous process of the eleventh thoracic vertebra? ( )

(1) Yishe (B 49)
(2) Jizhong (Du 6)
(3) Pishu (B 20)
(4) Yanggang (B 48)

34. Which of the following points is/are located at the level with the fourth intercostal space? ( )

(1) Tanzhong (Ren 17)
(2) Ruzhong (S 17)
(3) Zhejin (G 23)
(4) Yuanye (G 22)

35. Which of the following points is/are located 3 cun above the transverse crease of the wrist? ( )

(1) Zhigou (SJ 6)
(2) Huizong (SJ 7)
(3) Jianshi (P 5)
(4) Pianli (LI 6)

36. Which of the following points is/are located 5 cun above the transverse crease of the wrist? ( )

(1) Wenliu (LI 4)
(2) Sanyangluo (SJ 8)
(3) Ximen (P 4)
(4) Kongzui (L 6)

37. Which of the following points is/are at the level with Xinshu (B 15)? ( )

(1) Shendao (Du 11)
(2) Shenfeng (K 23)
(3) Shentang (UB 44)
(4) Shenmen (H 7)

38. Which of the following points is/are located 0.5 cun within the hairline? ( )

(1) Touwei (S 8)
(2) Shenting (Du 24)
(3) Benshen (G 13)
(4) Yamen (Du 15)

39. Which of the following points is/are located 5 cun above the malleolus? ( )

(1) Zhubin (K 9)
(2) Ligou (Liv 5)
(3) Guangming (GB 37)
(4) Lougu (Sp 7)

40. Which of the following points is/are located 3 cun above the malleolus? ( )

(1) Fuyang (UB 59)
(2) Xuanzong (G 39)
(3) Sanyinjiao (Sp 6)
(4) Fuliu (K 7)

41. Which of the following points is/are at the level with Shenting (Du 24)? ( )

(1) Benshen (G 13)
(2) Meichong (B 3)
(3) Toulinqi (G 15)
(4) Quchai (B 4)

42. Which of the following points is/are at the level with Yamen (Du 15)? ( )

(1) Fengchi (G 20)
(2) Fengfu (Du 16)

(3) Wangu (G 12)
(4) Tianzhu (B 10)

43. Which of the following points is/are contraindicated for both acupuncture and moxibustion? ( )

(1) Quepen (St 12)
(2) Shenque (Ren 8)
(3) Shimen (Ren 5)
(4) Ruzhong (S 17)

44. Which of the following points would you not use on a pregnant woman? ( )

(1) Quchi (LI 11)
(2) Hegu (LI 4)
(3) Yanglingquan (G 36)
(4) Sanyinjiao (Sp 6)

45. Which of the following statements is/are false? ( ).

(1) The "mother" point of the lung channel is Chize (Lu 5)
(2) The "mother" point of the large intestine channel is Quchi (LI 11)
(3) The "mother" point of the small intestine channel is Shaoze (SI 1)
(4) The "mother" point of the kidney channel is Fuliu (K 7)

46. Which of the following points is/are commonly used to cause bleeding? ( )

(1) Shixuan (Extra)
(2) Baxie (Extra)
(3) Sifeng (Extra)
(4) Sishencong (Extra)

47. The indications of Yinlingquan (Sp 9) are ( ).

(1) abdominal pain and distension, and diarrhea
(2) dysuria and edema
(3) enuresis and incontinence of urine
(4) pain in the knee

48. Which of the following points would you select to treat febrile diseases? ( )

(1) Dazhui (Du 14)
(2) Zhiyang (Du 19)
(3) Quchi (LI 11)
(4) Fengmen (B 12)

49. Which of the following points is/are not marked in Fig. 8? ( )

(1) Yangchi (SJ 4)
(2) Yanglao (SI 6)
(3) Waiguan (SI 5)
(4) Yangxi (LI 5)

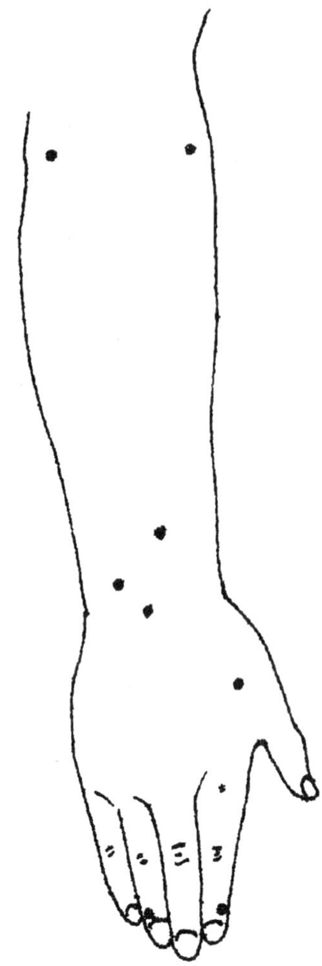

Fig. 8

50. Which of the following points is/are not marked in Fig. 9? ( )

(1) Sizhukong (SJ 22)
(2) Tongziliao (G 1)
(3) Quanliao (SI 18)
(4) Dicang (S 4)

51. Which of the following statements is/are true ( )

(1) The "mother" point of the lung channel is Chize (Lu 5)
(2) The "mother" point of the large intestine channel is Quchi (LI 11)
(3) The "mother" point of the small intestine channel is Shaoze (SI 1)
(4) The "mother" point of the kidney channel is Fuliu (K 7)

52. Which of the following statements regarding the "son" point is/are false? ( )

(1) The "son" point of the liver channel is Xingjian (Liv 2)
(2) The "son" point of the spleen channel is Shangqiu (Sp 5)
(3) The "son" point of the gallbladder channel is Yangfu (GB 38)
(4) The "son" point of the urinary bladder channel is Shugu (UB 65).

53. Channel(s) distributing to the tongue include(s) ( ).

(1) the liver channel
(2) the spleen channel
(3) the stomach channel
(4) the kidney channel

54. The point(s) for treating facial paralysis include ( ).

(1) Lingquan (Ren 23)

(2) Jiache (St 6)
(3) Shangxing (Du 26)
(4) Dicang (St 4)

55. The lower He-Sea points include ( ).
(1) the He points of the three Yang channels of the hand
(2) the He points of the three Yang channels of both hand and foot
(3) the He points of the three Yin channels of both hand and foot
(4) the He points of the three Yang channels of the foot

56. Which of the following statements regarding the attribution of the five-Shu points on yin Channels to the Five Elements is/are true? ( )
(1) the Jing-Well points relate to wood
(2) the He-Sea points relate to water
(3) the Shu-Stream points relate to earth
(4) the Xing-Spring points relate to fire

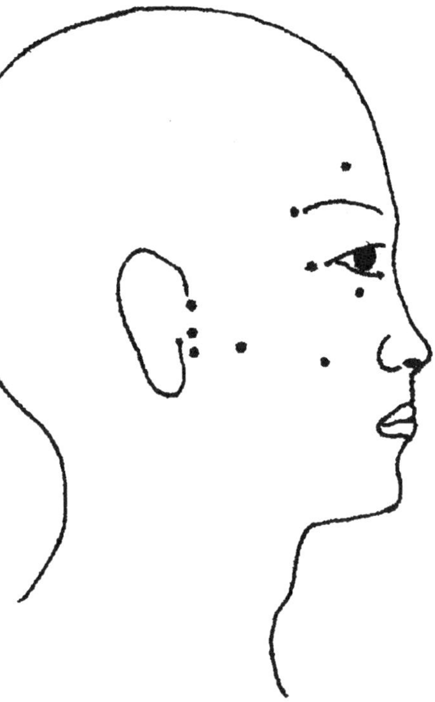

Fig. 9

IV. Diagnostic Methods

1. Red complexion indicates ( ).
(1) febrile diseases caused by exogenous pathogens
(2) excessive heat in the Zang-Fu organs
(3) deficient heat caused by a deficiency of yin
(4) floating of yang

2. Bluish purple complexion is due to ( ).
(1) stagnation of blood
(2) deficiency of blood
(3) severe pain

(4) stagnation of Qi

3. Pale complexion is linked with (   ).

(1) deficiency of blood
(2) deficiency of Qi
(3) deficiency of yang
(4) deficiency of yin

4. Pale complexion indicates (   ).

(1) deficient syndromes
(2) cold syndromes
(3) collapse of blood
(4) collapse of Qi

5. A normal tongue is (   ).

(1) proper size
(2) light red in colour
(3) free in motion
(4) thin white coating

6. A yellow complexion indicates (   ).

(1) heat syndromes
(2) damp syndromes
(3) wind syndromes
(4) deficiency syndromes

7. The tip of the tongue often reveals the pathological change of (   ).

(1) the heart
(2) the spleen
(3) the lung
(4) the stomach

8. A pale tongue indicates (   ).

(1) deficiency of Qi
(2) deficiency of blood
(3) deficiency of yang
(4) deficiency of yin

9. A red tongue indicates (   ).

(1) heat syndromes of the excessive type
(2) deficient blood syndromes
(3) heat syndromes of the deficient type

(4) deficient Qi shyndromes

10. A deep red tongue indicates ( ).

(1) extreme heat condition
(2) interior excess syndrome
(3) hyperactivity of fire due to deficient yin
(4) stagnation of blood

11. A pale purplish and moist tongue is related to ( ).

(1) extreme heat condition
(2) accumulation of cold
(3) deficiency of yin
(4) stagnation of blood

12. A blue purplish tongue, dry and lustreless, is related to ( ).

(1) stagnation of blood
(2) accumulation of cold
(3) extreme heat
(4) deficiency of yin

13. A swollen tongue indicates ( ).

(1) yang deficiency of the spleen and kidney
(2) retention of fluid, phlegm and dampness
(3) excess heat in the heart and spleen
(4) toxicosis

14. A cracked tongue indicates ( ).

(1) excess heat consuming body fluids
(2) deficiency of blood
(3) deficiency of Qi and yin
(4) invasion of pathogenic wind

15. A thin tongue indicates ( ).

(1) deficiency of yang
(2) deficiency of Qi and blood
(3) deficiency of the spleen
(4) deficiency of yin

16. The clinical significance of a deviated tongue is/are ( ).

(1) early signs of windstroke
(2) invasion of the heart by pathogenic heat
(3) windstroke

(4) sunstroke

17. The early signs of windstroke on the tongue is/are ( ).

(1) deviated
(2) flaccid
(3) rigid
(4) cracked

18. A rigid tongue indicates ( ).

(1) invasion of the pericardium by heat
(2) retention of turbid phlegm in the interior
(3) excessive pathogenic heat consuming body fluid
(4) windstroke

19. A white tongue coating indicates ( ).

(1) normal
(2) exterior syndromes
(3) cold syndromes
(4) damp syndromes

20. A white, thick and sticky tongue coating indicates ( ).

(1) retention of phlegm
(2) retention of undigested food
(3) retention of cold-damp
(4) stagnation of Qi

21. A dry tongue coating indicates ( ).

(1) deficiency of yin
(2) deficiency of body fluid
(3) deficiency of yang Qi which fails to transfer body fluid
(4) deficiency of blood

22. An obese patient with mental depression suggest ( ).

(1) deficiency of Qi
(2) deficiency of yang
(3) excess of phlegm-damp
(4) retention of food

23. Disturbance of the eye by liver wind may show ( ).

(1) upward staring
(2) straightforward staring
(3) sideways staring
(4) yellow sclera

24. Redness and swelling of the throat with yellow or white ulcer spots are due to excessive toxic heat in ( ).

(1) the heart
(2) the lung
(3) the spleen
(4) the stomach

25. Redness and swelling of the gums are due to a flare-up of ( ).

(1) heart fire
(2) lung fire
(3) spleen fire
(4) stomach fire

26. Blue purplish lips suggest ( ).

(1) retention of heat
(2) retention of cold
(3) stagnation of Qi
(4) stagnation of blood

27. Sweating is present in ( ).

(1) exterior syndromes
(2) interior syndromes
(3) deficient syndromes
(4) excessive syndromes

28. Profuse sweating caused by the total exhaustion of yang is often accompanied by ( ).

(1) listlessness
(2) feeble breathing
(3) cold limbs
(4) deep, thready pulse

29. The causes of spontaneous sweating include ( ).

(1) weakness of yang
(2) deficiency of yin
(3) deficiency of defensive Qi
(4) excessive heat

30. Spontaneous sweating is usually accompanied by ( ).

(1) listlessness
(2) lassitude
(3) worsening upon slight exertion

(4) afternoon fever

31. Night sweating caused by a deficiency of yin is usually accompanied by ( ).

(1) tidal fever
(2) chills
(3) a red tongue with little coating
(4) shortness of breath

32. The presence of thirst indicates ( ).

(1) deficiency of yang
(2) consumption of body fluid
(3) deficiency of Qi
(4) retention of phlegm-damp in the interior

33. Poor appetite caused by a weakness of the spleen and stomach is often accompanied by ( ).

(1) loose stools
(2) lassitude
(3) a pale tongue with a thin white coating
(4) sour regurgitation

34. Poor appetite due to a retention of pathogenic dampness is accompanied by ( ).

(1) stuffiness in the chest
(2) fullness in the abdomen
(3) thick sticky tongue coating
(4) soft pulse

35. Constipation due to dryness of the stools usually indicates ( ).

(1) retention of damp
(2) accumulation of heat
(3) deficiency of yang
(4) consumption of body fluid

36. Loose stools often suggest ( ).

(1) deficiency of the spleen
(2) stagnation of Qi
(3) retention of dampness
(4) retention of food

37. Clear urine with increased output indicates ( ).

(1) infirmity of kidney Qi

(2) retention of damp
(3) dysfunction of the bladder in controlling urine
(4) invasion of the bladder by heat.

38. Downward infusion of damp-heat into the bladder would cause ( ).
(1) scanty, yellow urine
(2) urgent urination
(3) painful urination
(4) enuresis

39. Dribbling urination is due to ( ).
(1) impaired function of the kidney for controlling urine
(2) Qi dysfunction inhibiting activities of the bladder due to downward infusion of the damp-heat
(3) stagnant blood or stones
(4) deficiency of yin

40. Retention of urine is usually caused by ( ).
(1) Qi dysfunction inhibiting the activities of the bladder due to downward infusion of damp-heat
(2) Qi dysfunction inhibiting the activities of the bladder due to downward infusion of stagnant blood
(3) Qi dysfunction inhibiting the activities of the bladder due to downward infusion of stones
(4) exhaustion of kidney Qi

41. The typical sign of pain caused by Qi stagnation is/are ( )
(1) a heavy sensation with pain
(2) distending pain
(3) burning pain
(4) pain moving from place to place

42. Headache may be caused by ( ).
(1) disturbance of the clear yang by the pathogens
(2) deficiency of Qi and blood which fails to nourish the head
(3) blockage of the channels by stagnation of Qi and blood
(4) retention of food

43. Lumbago may result from ( ).
(1) disturbance of the clear yang
(2) deficiency of the kidney
(3) retention of food

(4) obstruction of the channels

44. Chest pain indicates the pathologic changes of ( ).

(1) the heart
(2) the spleen
(3) the lung
(4) the kidney

45. Hypochondriac pain is linked with ( ).

(1) stagnation of Qi of the liver
(2) stagnation of blood of the liver
(3) damp-heat in the gallbladder
(4) damp-heat in the spleen

46. Epigastric pain may result from ( ).

(1) retention of food
(2) invasion of pathogenic cold
(3) deficiency of yang
(4) stagnation of liver Qi

47. Insomnia caused by a failure of the blood to nourish the heart and deficiency of both the heart and spleen is often accompanied by ( ).

(1) mental restlessness
(2) dizziness
(3) gastric discomfort
(4) palpitation

48. Insomnia due to hyperactivity of the fire of the heart is often accompanied by ( ).

(1) mental restlessness
(2) dizziness
(3) dream-disturbed sleep
(4) palpitation

49. Lethargy may result from ( ).

(1) deficiency of yin
(2) deficiency of yang
(3) stagnation of Qi
(4) accumulation of phlegm-damp in the interior

50. Excessive heat in the blood may result in menses ( ).

(1) of a shortened cycle

(2) being excessive in amount
(3) being deep red in colour
(4) being thick in quality

51. Stagnation of blood may result in ( ).
(1) a prolonged menstrual cycle
(2) low abdomen pain which intensifies on pressure
(3) scanty purplish-dark discharge or blood clots
(4) watery leukorrhea

52. A slow pulse (*chi mai*) indicates ( ).
(1) exterior syndrome
(2) interior syndrome
(3) heat syndrome
(4) cold syndrome

53. A rolling pulse (*hua mai*) indicates ( ).
(1) retention of phlegm
(2) retention of food
(3) excess heat
(4) pregnancy

54. A hesitant pulse (*se mai*) indicates ( ).
(1) deficiency of blood
(2) impairment of essence
(3) stagnation of Qi
(4) stagnation of blood

55. Pathogenic phlegm-damp may be reflected by ( ).
(1) a rolling pulse (*hua mai*)
(2) a string-taut pulse (*xuan mai*)
(3) a soft pulse (*ru mai*)
(4) a rapid pulse (*shuo mai*)

56. A string-taut pulse (*xuan mai*) indicates ( ).
(1) disorders of the liver and gallbladder
(2) painful syndromes
(3) retention of phlegm
(4) deficiency of yin

57. A thready pulse (xi mai) indicates ( ).
(1) deficiency of yin
(2) excess heat

(3) deficiency of Qi and blood
(4) spleen disease

58. The pulse which indicates a deficiency of both Qi and blood would be ( ).

(1) a thready pulse (*xi mai*)
(2) a weak pulse (*ruo mai*)
(3) a deficient pulse (*xu mai*)
(4) a slow pulse (*chi mai*)

59. Stagnation of blood results in ( ).

(1) immovable hard masses in the abdomen
(2) pain at definite site
(3) pricking pain
(4) a hesitant pulse (*se mai*)

60. A superficial and tense pulse (*fu* and *jin mai*) indicates ( ).

(1) exterior heat syndrome
(2) exterior deficient syndrome
(3) exterior damp syndrome
(4) exterior cold syndrome

61. A deviated tongue often indicates ( ).

(1) blood deficiency
(2) blood obstruction
(3) Qi deficiency
(4) obstruction of the channels and collaterals by wind-phlegm

62. Which of the following symptoms can be categorized as a sign of the lung channel? ( )

(1) sore throat
(2) pain in the supraclavicular fossa
(3) cough and asthma
(4) palpitation

63. The change in tongue proper that doesn't relate to heat syndrome includes ( ).

(1) red tongue
(2) purplish tongue
(3) deep red tongue
(4) pale tongue

64. Which of the following symptoms would be the most likely to help make

the diagnosis of invasion of the spleen by cold and dampness? ( ).

(1) distention in the epigastrium
(2) poor appetite
(3) heaviness of the head
(4) foul belching and sour regurgitation

65. Congested and sore throat can be seen in syndrome(s) of ( ).

(1) the lung channel
(2) the large intestine channel
(3) the kidney channel
(4) the urinary bladder channel

66. Retention of urine or difficult dribbling urination is often due to ( ).

(1) retention of damp-heat in the urinary bladder
(2) insufficiency of kidney yang
(3) presence of stones
(4) stagnant blood

67. Chills without fever may be caused by ( ).

(1) exogenous cold resulting from a deficiency of defensive Qi
(2) endogenous cold resulting from a deficiency of yang Qi
(3) invasion by wind-heat
(4) exogenous pathogenic cold directly effecting certain Zang-Fu organs

68. Might sweating is usually a sign indicating ( ).

(1) hyperactivity of yang
(2) excessive heat
(3) deficiency of yin
(4) exogenous pathogenic cold

69. Absence of thirst or thirst without desire to take fluids often indicates ( ).

(1) interior heat syndrome
(2) deficiency of yang Qi
(3) deficiency of yin
(4) cold-damp

70. A pale tongue (a less than normally red tongue) often indicates ( ).

(1) deficiency of Qi and blood
(2) deficiency of yin
(3) exogenous pathogenic cold
(4) deficiency of fluids

71. An abnormally red tongue often indicates ( ).

(1) cold
(2) pathogenic heat
(3) dampness
(4) yin deficiency

72. A deep red tongue often indicates ( ).

(1) pathogenic heat in the blood
(2) yin fluid has been exhausted and endogenous fire, which is of the deficiency type, is hyperactive
(3) pathogenic heat has been transmitted from the exterior to the interior of the body
(4) blood stasis

73. An enlarged tongue, which is pale in colour and has tooth-prints on the border, indicates ( ).

(1) deficiency of Qi
(2) deficiency of yang
(3) retention of phlegm-damp in the interior
(4) deficiency of blood

74. Irregular streaks or cracks on the tongue indicate ( ).

(1) consumption of body fluids by excessive heat
(2) hyperactivity of the fire due to a deficiency of yin
(3) loss of the essence of the kidney
(4) pathogenic dryness

V. Differentiation of Syndromes

1. The chief manifestation(s) of exterior syndromes is/are ( ).

(1) chills
(2) fever
(3) general aching
(4) thin tongue coating

2. The characteristics of exterior syndromes include ( ).

(1) sudden onset of symptoms with short duration
(2) chills and fever
(3) superficial pulse (*fu mai*)

(4) yellow tongue coating

3. The exterior syndromes are caused by (   ).

(1) traumatic injury
(2) phlegm and fluid in the lung
(3) deficiency of lung Qi
(4) invasion of the superficial portion of the body by exogenous pathogens

4. The causes of interior syndromes include (   ).

(1) emotional changes
(2) improper diet
(3) overstrain and stress
(4) invasion of the Zang-Fu organs by exogenous pathogens

5. Cold syndrome is often indicated by (   ).

(1) aversion to cold
(2) absence of thirst
(3) pallor
(4) slow pulse (*chi mai*)

6. Heat syndrome is usually indicated as (   ).

(1) thirst with preference for cold drinks
(2) yellow urine
(3) red tongue
(4) rapid pulse

7. The differentiation between exterior and interior syndromes can be made by (   ).

(1) pain or no pain
(2) sweating or no sweating
(3) cough or no cough
(4) fever with or without chills

8. The syndrome of true heat with false cold is suggested by (   ).

(1) cold limbs
(2) burning sensation in the chest and abdomen
(3) aversion to heat
(4) slow pulse (*chi mai*)

9. The syndrome of true cold with false heat is suggested by (   ).

(1) feverishness of the body
(2) flushed face

(3) preference for drinking warm drinks
(4) preference for heavy blankets

10. The syndrome of deficiency of yin results in ( ).
(1) afternoon fever
(2) night sweating
(3) malar flush
(4) heat sensation in the palms and soles

11. The manifestation(s) of a deficiency of yang include(s) ( ).
(1) chills
(2) spontaneous sweating
(3) clear urine with increased output
(4) slight tongue coating

12. the differentiation between a deficiency from the excess syndrome includes the following factors ( ).
(1) spirit
(2) strength of the voice and breath
(3) response to pressure on painful areas
(4) pulse

13. The manifestations of excess syndromes is/are ( ).
(1) coarse breathing
(2) lassitude
(3) pain aggravated by pressure
(4) disinclination to speak

14. The manifestation(s) of deficient syndromes include(s) ( ).
(1) listlessness
(2) lassitude
(3) feeble breathing
(4) sonorous voice

15. The manifestations of a deficiency of Qi include ( ).
(1) dizziness
(2) disinclination to speak
(3) lassitude
(4) thin red tongue

16. The clinical manifestations of a Qi-sinking syndrome include ( ).
(1) prolapse of the anus or uterus

(2) bearing-down, distending sensation in the abdominal region
(3) gastroptosis
(4) lassitude

17. The clinical manifestations of a Qi-stagnation syndrome include ( ).
(1) dizziness
(2) distention
(3) prolapse of the anus
(4) pain

18. The clinical manifestations of a deficiency-of-blood syndrome include ( ).
(1) pale lips
(2) palpitation
(3) numbness of the hands and feet
(4) insomnia

19. The clinical manifestations of a blood-stagnation syndrome include ( ).
(1) pain which is worse with pressure
(2) purplish spots on the tongue
(3) dark red menstrual flow with clots
(4) pale lips

20. The clinical manifestations of heat in the blood includes ( ).
(1) thready pulse (*xi mai*)
(2) hemorrhage
(3) palpitation
(4) mental restlessness

21. The clinical manifestations of heat in the blood include ( ).
(1) mental restlessness
(2) hemorrhage
(3) deep red tongue
(4) rapid pulse (*shuo mai*)

22. The syndrome of heat in the blood is often due to ( ).
(1) invasion of exogenous pathogenic heat
(2) deficiency of yin
(3) obstruction of liver Qi turning into fire
(4) stagnation of blood

23. The syndrome of deficiency of blood is often due to ( ).
(1) weakness of the spleen and stomach

(2) weakness of the lung
(3) excessive blood loss
(4) stagnation of Qi

24. The clinical manifestation(s) of a heart deficiency include ( ).
(1) palpitation
(2) shortness of breath
(3) lassitude
(4) chills

25. The clinical manifestation(s) of a heart yang deficiency include ( ).
(1) palpitation
(2) shortness of breath
(3) cold limbs
(4) pale, swollen tongue

26. The differentiation between a deficiency of heart yang from a deficiency of heart Qi can be made by the appearance of ( ).
(1) palpitaiton
(2) shortness of breath
(3) weak pulse (*ruo mai*)
(4) cold limbs

27. The clinical manifestation(s) of a deficiency of heart blood include(s) ( ).
(1) insomnia
(2) palpitation
(3) dizziness and vertigo
(4) thready and weak pulse (*xi* and *ruo mai*)

28. The clinical manifestations of a deficiency of heart yin include ( ).
(1) palpitation
(2) insomnia
(3) night sweating
(4) pale tongue

29. The differentiation between a deficiency of heart yin from a deficiency of heart blood can be made by the appearance of ( ).
(1) palpitation
(2) night sweating
(3) thready pulse (*xi mai*)
(4) red tongue

30. The clinical manifestations of a stagnation of heart blood include ( ).

(1) palpitation
(2) cardiac pain
(3) purplish spots on the tongue
(4) thready and weak pulse (*xi* and *ruo mai*)

31. The clinical manifestations of the syndrome of hyperactivity of heart fire include ( ).

(1) mental restlessness
(2) insomnia
(3) ulceration and pain of the tongue
(4) deep yellow urine

32. The clinical manifestations of "phlegm misting the heart" include ( )

(1) mental depression
(2) incoherent speech
(3) coma and gurgling with sputum in the throat
(4) violent behaviour

33. The clinical manifestations of "phlegm-fire disturbing the heart" include ( ).

(1) mental depression
(2) mania
(3) cardiac pain
(4) violent behaviour

34. Mania, violent behaviour, insomnia, dream-disturbed sleep, coarse breathing, deep-yellow urine, a yellow, sticky tongue coating and a rolling, rapid and forceful pulse (*hua*, *shuo* and *chi mai*) are due to the heart disturbed by ( ).

(1) cold
(2) damp
(3) wind
(4) phlegm

35. Mental depression and dullness or incoherent speech, weeping and coma and gurgling with sputum in the throat, a white, sticky tongue coating and a string-taut and rolling pulse (*xuan* and *hua mai*) are due to the heart disturbed by ( ).

(1) cold and dampness
(2) fire and dryness

(3) stagnation of heart blood
(4) phlegm

36. The clinical manifestation(s) of retention of phlegm-damp in the lung include ( ).

(1) cough with white sticky sputum
(2) fullness and stuffiness in the chest
(3) asthmatic breathing
(4) chills

37. The clinical manifestation(s) of retention of phlegm-heat in the lung may include ( ).

(1) cough
(2) yellow, thick sputum
(3) yellow, sticky tongue coating
(4) thirst

38. Cough, asthmatic and coarse breathing, yellow and thick sputum, chest pain upon coughing, yellow urine, a red tongue with a yellow, sticky coating and a rolling and rapid pulse (*hua* and *shuo mai*) may be caused by ( ).

(1) wind in the lung
(2) phlegm in the lung
(3) deficiency of lung yin
(4) heat in the lung

39. The clinical manifestation(s) of a deficiency of lung Qi include(s) ( ).

(1) feeble cough
(2) shortness of breath
(3) disinclination to speak
(4) low voice

40. Feeble cough, shortness of breath exacerbated upon exertion, lassitude, disinclination to speak, low voice, aversion to wind, spontaneous sweating, a pale tongue with a thin, white coating and a weak pulse (*ruo mai*) would suggest a diagnosis ( ).

(1) invasion of the lung by pathogenic wind
(2) retention of phlegm-damp in the lung
(3) deficiency of lung yin
(4) deficiency of lung Qi

41. The clinical manifestation(s) of an insufficiency of lung yin include(s) ( ).

(1) cough

(2) a sticky sputum
(3) afternoon fever
(4) night sweating

42. The clinical manifestation(s) of damp-heat in the large intestine include-(s) ( ).
(1) abdominal pain
(2) blood and mucus in the stools
(3) burning sensation of the anus
(4) a yellow, sticky tongue coating

43. The clinical manifestation(s) of a spleen-Qi deficiency include(s) ( ).
(1) loose stools
(2) decreased appetite
(3) abdominal distention
(4) yellow urine

44. The differentiation between a deficiency of spleen yang and a deficiency of spleen Qi can be made by ( ).
(1) loose stools
(2) cold limbs
(3) a pale tougue with a white coating
(4) a deep, slow pulse (*chen* and *chi mai*)

45. The clinical manifestation(s) of a spleen-yang deficiency include(s) ( ).
(1) loose stools
(2) cold limbs
(3) poor appetite
(4) a pale tongue and a deep, slow pulse (*chen* and *chi mai*)

46. Fullness and distention in the epigastrium and abdomen, decreased appetite, nausea, vomiting, bitter taste and stickiness of the mouth, heaviness of the body, lassitude, bright yellow face, eyes and skin, loose stools, scanty and yellow urine, and a yellow, sticky tongue coating with a soft, rapid pulse (*ru* and *shuo mai*) indicates a spleen and stomach syndrome caused by ( ).
(1) dampness
(2) retention of food
(3) deficiency of spleen yang
(4) damp-heat

47. Fullness and distention in the epigastrium and abdomen, decreased appetite, sticky saliva, heaviness of the head and body, loose stools or

diarrhea, a white, sticky tongue coating with a soft pulse (*ru mai*) results from a/an ( ).

(1) insufficiency of stomach yin
(2) deficiency of spleen Qi
(3) retention of food in the stomach
(4) invasion of the spleen by cold-damp

48. Distention, fullness and pain in the epigastrium and abdomen, foul belching and sour regurgitation, anorexia, a thick and sticky tongue coating, and a rollin g pulse (*hua mai*) results from a/an ( ).

(1) hyperactivity of fire in the stomach
(2) retention of fluid in the stomach due to cold
(3) retention of fluid in the stomach
(4) retention of food in the stomach

49. Burning sensation and pain in the epigastric region, sour regurgitation and an empty and uncomfortable feeling in the stomach, thirst with preference for cold drinks, voracious appetite and getting hungry easily, vomiting, foul breath, swelling and pain or ulceration and bleeding of the gums, constipation, scanty yellow urine, a red tongue with a yellow coating and a rapid pulse (*shuo mai*) results from a/an ( ).

(1) retention of food in the stomach
(2) retention of fluid in the stomach due to cold
(3) insufficiency of stomach yin
(4) hyperactivity of fire in the stomach

50. The clinical manifestations of an insufficiency of stomach yin include ( ).

(1) burning pain in the epigastric region
(2) constipation
(3) hunger
(4) no desire to eat

51. The clinical manifestations of a dysfunction of the spleen in controlling blood include ( ).

(1) pale complexion
(2) bloody stools
(3) thready, weak pulse (*xi* and *ruo mai*)
(4) red tongue

52. The clinical manifestations of a stagnation of liver Qi include ( ).

(1) mental depression

(2) pain in the costal and hypochondriac regions
(3) abdominal distension
(4) distension of the breasts

53. Irregular menstruation, distention of the breasts, mental depression, a thin , white tongue coating with a string-taut pulse (*xuan mai*) indicate ( ).

(1) deficiency of heart blood
(2) deficiency of kidney yang
(3) deficiency of spleen Qi
(4) stagnation of liver Qi

54. The clinical manifestations of damp-heat in the liver and gallbladder include ( ).

(1) yellow, sclera and skin over the entire body
(2) bitter taste in the mouth
(3) scanty and yellow urine
(4) yellow, sticky tongue coating

55. Yellow, sclera and skin over the entire body, fever, bitter taste in the mouth, hypochondriac distention, decreased appetite, nausea, vomiting, scanty and yellow urine, a yellow, sticky tongue coating with a string-taut, and rapid pulse (*xuan* and *shuo mai*) are caused by damp-heat in ( ).

(1) the liver
(2) the bladde
(3) the gallbladder
(4) the stomach

56. The clinical manifestations of a deficiency of kidney Qi include ( ).

(1) soreness and weakness of the lumbar region and knee joints
(2) dribbling of urine after urination
(3) frequent urination with clear urine
(4) cold limbs

57. The differentiation between an insufficiency of kidney yang and a deficiency of kidney Qi is ( ).

(1) soreness and weakness of the lumbar region and knee joints
(2) frequent urination with clear urine
(3) dizziness
(4) cold limbs

58. The clinical manifestations of an insufficiency of kidney yang are ( ).

(1) soreness and weakness of the lumbar region and knee joints

(2) impitence
(3) dizziness
(4) cold limbs

59. The clinical manifestations of damp-heat in the bladder include ( ).
(1) frequency and urgency of urination
(2) burning pain in the urethra
(3) deep yellow urine
(4) yellow sclera and skin

60. The clinical manifestations of an invasion of the lung by liver fire include ( ).
(1) burning pain in the costal and hypochondriac regions
(2) paroxysmal cough
(3) bitter taste in the mouth
(4) red tongue with yellow coating

61. The clinical manifestations of a disharmony between the heart and kidney include ( ).
(1) insomnia
(2) palpitation
(3) soreness of the lumbar region
(4) tinnitus

VI. Techniques of Acupuncture, Moxibustion and Cupping

1. In clinic the depth of insertion of a needle depends upon ( ).
(1) the constitution of the patient
(2) the location of the point
(3) the pathological condition
(4) the length of the needle

2. Which of the following point(s) is/are often needled obliquely? ( ).
(1) Lieque (L 7)
(2) Pianli (LI 6)
(3) Qimen (Liv 14)
(4) Xingjian (Liv 2)

3. Which of the following point(s) is/are often needled horizontally? ( )
(1) Baihui (Du 20)

(2) Touwei (S 8)
(3) Zanzhu (B 2)
(4) Tanzhong (Ren 17)

4. The sign(s) of the arrival of Qi may include(s) ( ).
(1) soreness
(2) numbness
(3) heaviness
(4) distention

5. The factor(s) influencing the arrival of Qi include(s) ( ).
(1) location of the points
(2) the depth of needle insertion
(3) needle manipulation
(4) constitution and sensation of the patient

6. Stuck needle may be caused by ( ).
(1) strong spasm of the local muscle after the insertion of the needle
(2) twirling the needle with too large amplitude
(3) twirling the needle in one direction only
(4) poor quality of the needle

7. Bent needle may result from ( ).
(1) unskillful manipulation or too forceful manipulation
(2) the needle striking the hard tissue
(3) a sudden change of the patient's posture
(4) twirling the needle with too large amplitude

8. The indication(s) of the three-edged needle is/are ( ).
(1) high fever
(2) loss of consciousness
(3) sore throat
(4) local congestion or swelling

9. The function(s) of the three-edged needle is/are ( ).
(1) to promote the smooth flow of Qi and blood in channels
(2) to dispel blood stasis
(3) to eliminate the heat
(4) to reinforce the deficiency

10. The cupping method has the function of ( ).
(1) warming

(2) promoting the free flow of Qi and blood
(3) dispelling cold-damp
(4) diminishing swelling and pain

11. Which of the following needling techniques belongs to the reinforcing method ? (   )

(1) lifting the needle gently and slowly
(2) rotating the needle gently and slowly with small amplitude
(3) inserting the needle slowly and withdrawing it rapidly
(4) pressing the hole quickly to close it after withdrawing the needle

12. The function(s) of moxibustion is/are (   ).

(1) to warm the channels and expel cold
(2) to induce the smooth flow of Qi and blood
(3) to strengthen yang from collapse
(4) to prevent diseases and maintain healthy

13. moxibusiton with ginger can be used to treat (   ).

(1) weakness of the stomach and spleen
(2) invasion of heat
(3) yang deficiency
(4) yin deficiency

14. An appropriate posture is selected for a patient according to (   ).

(1) the location of the points utilized
(2) the manipulation utilized for acupuncture and moxibustion treatment
(3) the duration the needles are retaind for a treatment
(4) the position best able to prevent fainting, bent needle, stuck needle or broken needle

15. Which of the following points is/are commonly used for moxibustion with salt (   ).

(1) Dazhui (Du 14)
(2) Zusanli (S 36)
(3) Sanyinjiao (Sp 6)
(4) Shenque (Ren 8)

16. The function(s) of moxibustion on ginger include(s) (   ).

(1) clearing pathogenic heat
(2) dispersing cold
(3) detoxification
(4) warming the middle Jiao

VII. Treatment of Diseases

1. The ascending treatment method would not be used for patients with ( ).

(1) sinking of the Qi in the middle Jiao
(2) prolapse of the rectum
(3) prolonged dysentery
(4) hyperactivity of yang due to a yin deficiency

2. Which of the following points is/are commonly used for soothing the liver and subduing liver yang? ( ).

(1) Fengchi (G 20)
(2) Taichong (Liv 3)
(3) Yongquan (K 1)
(4) Zhongwan (Ren 12)

3. Which of the following points is/are often utilized with the clearing method? ( )

(1) Dazhui (Du 14)
(2) Quchi (LI 11)
(3) Hegu (LI 4)
(4) Yamen (Du 15)

4. Which of the following points is/are often utilized for clearing heat and resuscitation? ( )

(1) Renzhong (Du 26)
(2) Dazhui (Du 14)
(3) the twelve Jing-Well points
(4) the confluent points of the eight extra meridians (or channels)

5. Which of the following groups of points pertains to the combination of the Yuan-Primary point and the Luo-Connecting point? ( )

(1) Hegu (LI 4)-Wenliu (LI 7)
(2) Daling (P7-Huizong (SJ 7)
(3) Shenmen (H 7)- Yanglao (SI 6)
(4) Taichong (Liv 3)-Guangming (G 37)

6. Which of the following points is/are Front-Mu point(s)? ( )

(1) Shangwan (Ren 13)
(2) Riyue (G 24)
(3) Qugu (Ren 2)
(4) Juque (Ren 14)

7. Which of the following points is/are Front-Mu point(s)? ( )

(1) Jingmen (G 25)
(2) Liangmen (St 21)
(3) Zhongfu (L 1)
(4) Qihai (Ren 6)

8. Which of the following points is/are Xi-Cleft point(s)? ( )

(1) Kongzui (L 6)
(2) Wenliu (LI 7)
(3) Jingmen (B 63)
(4) Fuyang (B 59)

9. Which of the following points is/are Luo-connecting point(s) as well as confluent point(s) of the eight extra meridians? ( )

(1) Zhaohai (K 6)
(2) Waiguan (SJ 5)
(3) Houxi (SI 3)
(4) Gongsun (Sp 4)

10. According to the functions of the eight confluent points, Houxi (SI 3) and Shenmai (B 62) can be combined together to treat the disorders of ( ).

(1) the inner canthus
(2) retroauricle region
(3) neck, shoulders and back
(4) throat and chest

11. In the eight confluent points of the eight extra meridians, the combination of Waiguan (SJ 5) with Zulinqi (G 41) can be used to treat the disorders of ( ).

(1) the heart, chest and stomach
(2) the neck, shoulder, back and inner canthus
(3) the throat, chest and lung
(4) the retroauricle region, cheek and outer canthus

12. Zusanli (S 36) is one of ( ).

(1) the lower He-Sea points
(2) the eight confluent points
(3) the five Shu points
(4) the eight influential points

13. According to the principle of selecting the "mother point" for reinforcing and the "son point" for reducing, which of the following points can be

needled for a case of fullness in the chest, restlessness, cough, yellow, thick sputum with a rapid, rolling pulse (*shuo* and *hua mai*)? (   )

(1) Taiyuan (L 9)
(2) Chize (L 5)
(3) Taibai (Sp 3)
(4) Yingu (K 10)

14. According to the principle of selecting the "mother point" for deficiency syndromes, and the "son point" for excess syndromes, which of the following points would you select first for a case of dizziness and vertigo, redness, swelling and pain of the eyes, a bitter taste and dryness in the mouth, burning pain i n the costal and hypochondriac regions, a red tongue with a yellow coating and a string-taut, rapid pulse (*xuan* and *shuo mai*) (   ).

(1) Dadun (Liv 1)
(2) Yingu (K 10)
(3) Taichong (Liv 3)
(4) Xingjian (Liv 2)

15. Which of the following point(s) would you select first for night sweating? (   )

(1) Dazhui (Du 14)
(2) Houxi (SI 3)
(3) Neiguan (P 6)
(4) Yinxi (H 6)

16. Which of the following point(s) is/are frequently selected for the treatment of hypochondrium pain? (   )

(1) Zhigou (SJ 6)
(2) Hegu (LI 4)
(3) Yanglingquan (G 34)
(4) Ximen (P 4)

17. Which of the following points is/are frequently selected for the treatment of fever? (   )

(1) Dazhui (Du 14)
(2) Hegu (LI 4)
(3) Quchi (LI 11)
(4) Zhigou (SJ 6)

18. Shenting (Du 24) is the crossing point of (   ).

(1) Hand-Taiyang meridian

(2) Foot-Taiyang meridian
(3) Foot-Shaoyang meridian
(4) Foot-Yangming meridian

19. Dazhui (Du 14) is the crossing point of ( ).
(1) Foot-Taiyang meridian
(2) Foot-Shaoyang meridian
(3) Foot-Yangming meridian
(4) Hand-Yangming meridian

20. Bingfeng (SI 12) is the crossing point of ( ).
(1) Foot-Shaoyang meridian
(2) Hand-Shaoyang meridian
(3) Foot-Yangming meridian
(4) Hand-Yangming meridian

21. Besides Shuigou (Du 26) and the twelve Jing-Well points, which of the following points would you select first for treating a tense syndrome of wind stroke? ( )
(1) Taichong (Liv 3)
(2) Fenglong (S 40)
(3) Yongquan (K 1)
(4) Qihai (Ren 6)

22. Which of the following points woulod be used for treating a case of chills, fever, headache, soreness and pain of the limbs, nasal obstruction, running nose, a thin white tongue coating and a superficial and tense pulse (*fu* and *jin mai*)? ( )
(1) Fengfu (Du 16), Fengmen (B 12), Fengchi (G 20)
(2) Taixi (K 3), Shenshu (B 23)
(3) Lieque (L 7), Hegu (LI 4)
(4) Yuji (L 10), Shousanli (LI 10)

23. Which of the following points would be selected to treat a case of fever, sweating, aversion to wind, headache, cough with yellow, thick sputum, sore throat , thirst, a thin, yellow tongue coating, and a superficial, rapid pulse (*fu* and *shuo mai*)? ( )
(1) Shaoshang (L 11), Yuji (L 10)
(2) Dazhui (Du 14)
(3) Quchi (LI 11), Hegu (LI 4)
(4) Waiguan (SJ 5)

24. Which of the following points can be used to treat a patient with the following signs and symptoms: cough, profuse, white and sticky sputum, stuffiness and depressed feeling of the chest, lack of appetite, a white, sticky tongue coating with a rolling pulse (*hua mai*)? ( )

(1) Feishu (B 13), Zhongwan (Ren 12)
(2) Chize (L 5)
(3) Zusanli (S 36), Fenglong (S 40)
(4) Zhaohai (K 6)

25. Which of the following points can be used to treat a patient with the following signs and symptoms: dry cough, no sputum, dryness of the nose and throat, sore throat, malar flush, red tongue with a thin coating, and a thready and rapid pulse (*xi* and *shuo mai*)? ( )

(1) Feishu (B 13), Zhongfu (L 1)
(2) Zhongwan (Ren 12), Fenglong (S 40)
(3) Lieque (L 7), Zhaohai (K 6)
(4) Hegu (LI 4), Quchi (LI 11)

26. Which of the following points can be used to treat a patient with the following signs and symptoms: short and rapid breathing, feeble voice, a cough with weak and low sound, sweating upon exertion, a plae tongue and a deficient pulse (*xu mai*)? ( )

(1) Feishu (B 13)
(2) Taiyuan (L 9)
(3) Zusanli (S 36)
(4) Taichong (Liv 3)

27. Which of the following points can be used to treat a patient with the following signs and symptoms: paroxysmal pain in the epigastrium which radiates to the hypochondrium, frequent belching accompanied by nausea, vomiting, acid regurgitation, abdominal distention, anorexia, a thin, white tongue coating and a deep, string-taut pulse (*chen* and *xuan mai*)? ( )

(1) Qimen (Liv 14), Taichong (Liv 3)
(2) Zusanli (S 36), Zhongwan (Ren 12)
(3) Neiguan (P 6)
(4) Pishu (B 20), Taixi (K 3)

28. Which of the following pairs of points would you select to treat a patient with the following signs and symptoms: intermittent dull abdominal pain which may be relieved by warmth or pressure and is aggravated by cold,

hunger, and fatigue, lassitude, aversion to cold, thin, white tongue coating and a deep, thready pulse (*chen* and *xi mai*)? ( )

(1) Pishu (B 20), Weishu (B 21)
(2) Zhongwan (Ren 12), Qihai (Ren 6)
(3) Zhangmen (Liv 13), Zusanli (St 36)
(4) Neiguan (P 6), Taichong (Liv 3)

29. Which of the following points owuld you select to treat a patient with the following signs and symptoms: diarrhea, abdominal pain, yellow, hot and fetid stools, burning sensation in the anus, scanty urine, desire for fluid, a yellow, sticky tongue coating and a rolling, rapid pulse (*hua* and *shuo mai*)? ( )

(1) Tianshu (S 25)
(2) Mingmen (Du 4), Guanyuan (Ren 4)
(3) Neiting (S 44), Yinlingquan (Sp 9)
(4) Zhongwan (Ren 12), Taibai (Sp 3)

30. Which of the following points can you select to treat a patient with the following signs and symptoms: yellow skin and sclera, fever, desire for fluids, scanty dark-yellow urine, heaviness of the body, fullness in the abdomen, stuffiness of the chest, nausea, a yellow, sticky tongue coating, and a string-taut, rapid pulse (*xuan* and *shuo mai*)? ( )

(1) Yinlingquan (Sp 9), Zusanli (S 36)
(2) Ganshu (B 18), Danshu (B 19)
(3) Zhiyang (Du 9)
(4) Taichong (Liv 3), Yanglingquan (G 34)

31. Points on which of the following channel's can be selected to treat edema? ( )

(1) the lung channel
(2) the spleen channel
(3) the kidney channel
(4) the Sanjiao channel

32. Which of the following point(s) can be selected to treat constipation? ( )

(1) Dachangshu (B 25)
(2) Tianshu (S 25)
(3) Zhigou (SJ 6)
(4) Zhaohai (K 6)

33. Which of the following point(s) can be selected to treat prolapse of the

rectum? ( )

(1) Baihui (Du 20)
(2) Dachangshu (B 25)
(3) Changqiang (Du 1)
(4) Zusanli (S 36)

34. Which of the following points are selected to treat a patient with the following signs and symptoms: imotence, bitter taste in the mouth, desire for fluids, hot and dark-red urine, a yellow, sticky tongue coating, and a soft, rapid pulse (*shuo* and *ruo mai*)? ( )

(1) Guanyuan (Ren 4), Mingmen (Du 4)
(2) Zhongji (Ren 3), Sanyinjiao (Sp 6)
(3) Shenshu (B 23), Taixi (K 3)
(4) Yinlingquan (Sp 9), Zusanli (S 36)

35. Which of the following points are selected to treat a patient with the following signs and symptoms: insomnia, dizziness, tinnitus, burning sensation in the chest, palms and soles, palpitation, lower back pain, a red tongue, and a thready rapid pulse (*xi* and *shuo mai*)? ( )

(1) Shenmen (H 7), Sanyinjiao (Sp 6), Anmian (Extra)
(2) Ganshu (B 16), Danshu (B 19), Wangu (G 12)
(3) Xinshu (B 15), Shenshu (B 23), Taixi (K 3)
(4) Weishu (B 21), Zusanli (S 36)

36. Which of the following points can be selected to treat pain at the maxillary region? ( )

(1) Sibai (S 2), Quanliao (SI 18)
(2) Yangbai (G 14), Zanzhu (B 2)
(3) Yingxiang (LI 20), Hegu (LI 4)
(4) Jiache (S 6), Jiachengjiang (Extra 8)

37. Which of the following points should be selected to treat lower back pain? ( )

(1) Shenshu (B 23)
(2) Yaoyangguan (B 23)
(3) Weizhong (B 40)
(4) Sanyinjiao (Sp 6)

38. Which of the following points should be selected to treat a patient with the following signs and symptoms: profuse, thin and light-red menses in shortened cycle, lassitude, palpitation, shortness of breath, pale tongue with

a thin coating, and a weak pulse (Xu mai)? ( )

(1) Xuehai (Sp 10), Quchi (LI 11)
(2) Qihai (Ren 6), Zhongwan (Ren 12)
(3) Xingjian (Liv 2), Zhongji (Ren 13)
(4) Sanyinjiao (Sp 6), Zusanli (S 36)

39. Which of the following points can be selected to treat a patient with the following signs and symptoms: dysmenorrhea usually starting before menstruation, delayed and scanty, dark-purple menses with clots, distending pain in the lower abdomen (alleviated by passing clots), distention in the hypochondrium and breast, a purplish tongue with purple spots on its edge, deep and a string-taut pulse (*chen* and *xuan mai*)? ( )

(1) Zhongji (Ren 3), Ciliao (B 32)
(2) Hegu (LI 4), Xuehai (Sp 10)
(3) Diji (Sp 8), Taichong (Liv 3)
(4) Guanyuan (Ren 4), Shenshu (B 23)

40. Which of the following points should be selected to treat a patient with the following signs and symptoms: continuous scanty uterine bleeding marked by light red and thin blood, lassitude, shortness of breath, apathy, anorexia, loose stools, pale tongue, and a weak, thready pulse (*xi* and *ruo mai*)? ( )

(1) Baihui (Du 20), Guanyuan (Ren 4)
(2) Zusanli (S 36), Sanyinjiao (Sp 6)
(3) Yinbai (Sp 1), Yangchi (SJ 4)
(4) Pishu (B 20), Weishu (B 21)

41. Which of the following points should be selected to treat a patient with the following signs and symptoms: profuse, white vaginal odourless discharge, pale complexion, lassitude, poor appetite, loose stools, edema of the lower limbs, a pale tongue with a white, sticky coating, and a slow, weak pulse (*chi* and *ruo mai*)? ( )

(1) Daimai (B 26), Qihai (Ren 6), Baihuanshu (B 30)
(2) Shenshu (B 23), Guanyuan (Ren 4), Fuliu (K 7)
(3) Yinlingquan (Sp 9), Zusanli (S 36)
(4) Zhongji (Ren 3), Taichong (Liv 3)

42. Which of the following points are selected to treat breast abscess? ( )

(1) Jianjing (G 21), Tanzhong (Ren 17)
(2) Rugen (S 18), Shaoze (SI 1)
(3) Zusanli (S 36), Taichong (Liv 3)

(4) Hegu (LI 4), Waiguan (SJ 5)

43. Which of the following points are selected to treat insufficientlactation? ( )

(1) Rugen (S 28)
(2) Tanzhong (Ren 17)
(3) Shaoze (SI 1)
(4) Taichong (Liv 3)

44. Which of the following points are selected to treat toothache caused by wind -fire? ( )

(1) Fengchi (G 20), Hegu (LI 4)
(2) Jiache (S 6), Xiaguan (S 7)
(3) Waiguan (SJ 5)
(4) Taixi (K 3), Xingjian (Liv 2)

Solutions to the Exercises

I.

1. B; 2. A; 3. A; 4. C; 5. A; 6. E; 7. A; 8. B; 9. C; 10. E; 11. A; 12. E; 13. B ; 14. C; 15. C; 16. B; 17. B; 18. D; 19. C; 20. B.

II.

1. B; 2. A; 3. E; 4. D; 5. E; 6. C; 7. E; 8. A; 9. E; 10. B; 11. E; 12. C; 13. B ; 14. C; 15. E; 16. B; 17. A; 18. D; 19. E; 20. E; 21. A; 22. E; 23. E; 24. B; 2 5. C; 26. E; 27. A; 28. C; 29. A; 30. E; 31. A; 32. A; 33. D; 34. C; 35. E; 36. E; 37. A; 38. A; 39. A; 40. E; 41. A; 42. D; 43. D; 44. A; 45. E.

III.

1. B; 2. A; 3. E; 4. A; 5. C; 6. A; 7. E; 8. B; 9. A; 10. A; 11. B; 12. A; 13. E ; 14. A; 15. B; 16. A; 17. B; 18. D; 19. C; 20. D; 21. A; 22. B; 23. D; 24. C; 2 5. A; 26. A; 27. E; 28. A; 29. A; 30. E; 31. E; 32. E; 33. A; 34. E; 35. E; 36. B; 37. B; 38. E; 39. A; 40. A; 41. E; 42. D; 43. D; 44. C; 45. B; 46. A; 47. E; 48. B; 49. C; 50. D; 51. C; 52. E; 53. C; 54. C; 55. D; 56. E.

IV.

1. E; 2. B; 3. A; 4. E; 5. E; 6. C; 7. B; 8. A; 9. B; 10. B; 11. C; 12. B; 13. E ; 14. A; 15. C; 16. B; 17. B; 18. E; 19. A; 20. A; 21. A; 22. A; 23. A; 24. C; 2 5. D; 26. C; 27. E; 28. E; 29. B; 30. A; 31. B; 32. C; 33. A; 34. E; 35. C; 36. B; 37. B; 38. A; 39. A; 40. E; 41. C; 42. A; 43. C; 44. B; 45. A; 46. E; 47. C; 48. B; 49. C; 50. E; 51. A; 52. D; 53. E; 54. E; 55. A; 56. A; 57. A; 58. A; 59. E; 60. D; 61. D; 62. A; 63. C; 64. A; 65. A; 66. E; 67.

C; 68. A; 69. D; 70. B; 71. C; 72. A; 73. A; 74. A.

V.

1. E; 2. A; 3. D; 4. E. 5. E; 6. E; 7. D; 8. A; 9. E; 10. E; 11. A; 12. E; 13. B ; 14. A; 15. A; 16. E; 17.C; 18. E; 19. A; 20. C; 21. E; 22. B; 23. B; 24. A; 25 . E; 26. D; 27. E; 28. A; 29. C; 30. A; 31. E; 32. A; 33. C; 34. D; 35. D; 36. A ; 37. A; 38. C; 39. E; 40. D; 41. E; 42. E; 43. A; 44. C; 45. E; 46. D; 47. C; 4 8. D; 49. D; 50. E; 51. A; 52. E; 53. D; 54. E; 55. B; 56. A; 57. D; 58. E; 59. A; 60. E; 61. E.

VI.

1. A; 2. E; 3. E; 4. E; 5. E; 6. A; 7. A; 8. E; 9. A; 10. E; 11. E; 12. E; 13. B ; 14. E; 15. D; 16. C.

VII.

1. D; 2. A; 3. A; 4. B; 5. D; 6. C; 7. B; 8. E; 9. C; 10. B; 11. D; 12. B; 13. C ; 14. D; 15. C; 16. B; 17. A; 18. C; 19. A; 20. E; 21. A; 22. B; 23. E; 24. A; 2 5. B; 26. A; 27. A; 28. A; 29. B; 30. E; 31. E; 32. E; 33. E; 34. C; 35. B; 36. B; 37. A; 38. C; 39. A; 40. E; 41. B; 42. A; 43. A; 44. A

Part Two Traditional Questions

I. Underline the Part of the Statement Which Is Incorrect

Example:
Chengqi (St 1) is indicated in patients with dysopia, <u>abdominal pain,</u> headache and blurred vision.

1. Daling (P 7) is indicated in patients with lumbar pain, abdominal pain and abdominal distention.

2. Dazhui (Du 14) is indicated in patients with a fever, malaria, asthma, epigastric pain and neck rigidity.

3. Tiantu (Ren 22) is indicated in patients with asthma, chest pain, abdominal pain, belching and hiccups.

4. Baihui (Du 20) is indicated in patients with a headache, mania, lumbar pain, facial paralysis and prolapse of the uterus.

5. Yanglingquan (GB 34) is indicated in patients with numbness and pain of the lower extremities, hypochondriac pain, cough, vomitting, and a bitter taste in the mouth.

6. Fengfu (Du 16) is indicated in patients with post-apoplexy aphasia, sore throat, headache and diarrhea.

7. Zhiyin (UB 67) is indicated in patients with difficult labour, headache, nasal obstruction and constipation.

8. Neiguan (P 6) is indicated in patients with cardiac pain, vomiting, cough, insomnia and mania.

9. Zhongzhu (SJ 3) is indicated in patients with tinnitus, deafness, headache, lumbar pain and soreness in the elbow.

10. Sanyinjiao (Sp 6) is indicated in patients with menstrual disorders, insomnia,

cardiac pain and abdominal distension.

11. Tianzhu (UB 10) is indicated in patients with appendicitis, diarrhea, hypochondrium pain and constipation.

12. Zanzhu (UB 2) is indicated in patients with red eyes, headache, toothache and pain in the supraorbital region.

13. Quchi (LI 11) is indicated in patients with urticaria, fever, mania, palpitation and a toothache.

14. Neiting (St 44) is indicated in patients with cough, toothache, stomachache, diarrhea and abdominal distention.

15. Waiguan (SJ 5) is indicated in patients with arm and wrist pair, malaria, dysentery and a common cold.

16. Fengchi (GB 20) is indicated in patients with headache, neck rigidity, dysentery, common cold and tinnitus.

17. Taibai (Sp 3) is indicated in patients with stomachache, sunstroke, abdominal distention, constipation and diarrhea.

18. Shenmen (H 7) is indicated in patients with insomnia, palpitation, lumbar sprain and a cough.

19. Taichong (Liv 13) is indicated in patients with headache, blurred vision, edema and enuresis.

Solutions to the Exercises

1. lumbar pain; 2. epigastric pain; 3. abdominal pain; 4. facial paralysis; 5. cough; 6. diarrhea; 7. constipation; 8. cough; 9. lumbar pain; 10. cardiac pain and abdominal distension; 11. hypochondrium pain; 12. toothache; 13. palpitation; 14. cough; 15. dysentery; 16. dysentery; 17. sunstroke; 18. lumbar sprain and a cough; 19. edema and enuresis.

II. True of False

If the statement is true, fill in the blank with the letter "T"; if the statement is false, fill in the blank with the letter "F".

1. Qiaoyin (GB 44) is the Jing-Well point of the gallbladder channel. ( )

Zulinqi (GB 41) is the Ying-Spring point of the gallbladder channel. ( )
Xiaxi (GB 43) is the Shu-Stream point of the gallbladder channel. ( )
Xuanzhong (GB 39) is the Jing-River point of the gallbladder channel. ( )
Yanglingquan (GB 34) is the He -Sea point of the gallbladder channel. ( )
2. Dadu (Sp 2) is the Yuan-Source point of the spleen channel. ( )
Gongsun (Sp 4) is the Luo-Connecting point of the spleen channel. ( )
3. Kunlun (B 60) is the Yuan-Source point of the urinary bladder channel. ( )
4. Feiyang (UB 58) is the Jing-river point of the urinary bladder channel. ( )
5. The Xi-Cleft point of the pericardium channel is Neiguan (P 6). ( )
6. The Xi-Cleft point of the Yinqiao channel is Jiaoxin (K 8). ( )
7. Shousanli (LI 10) is located 2 cun below Quchi (LI 11). ( )
8. Zhubin (K 9) is located 6 cun above Taixi (K 3). ( )
9. Liangmen (St 21) is located 2 cun lateral to Zhongwan (Ren 12). ( )
10. Zhangmen (Liv 13) is located at the free end the twelfth floating rib. ( )
11. Yingu (K 10) is located on the lower border of the medial condyle of the tibia. ( )
12. Xiaguan (St 7) is in the depression at the lower border of the zygomatic arch. ( )
13. Guanyuan (Ren 4) and Yongquan (K 1) are points which are often utilized for tonification. ( )
14. The distance between the centre of the patella and the tip of the lateral malleolus is 13 cun. ( )
15. Yangxi (LI 5) is the Luo-Connecting point of the large intestine channel. ( )
16. Xuanzhong (G 39) is the Luo-Connecting point of the gallbladder channel. ( )
17. The extraordinary point Sifeng (Extra 25) is mainly used in treating common colds in infants. ( )
18. The extraordinary point Dannangxue (Extra 39) is utlized for acute and chronic cholecystitis. ( )
19. The points Yangbai (G 14), Zanzhu (UB 2), Dicang (St 4) and Hegu (LI 4) are effective in treating facial paralysis. ( )
20. The three yin channels of the hand run from the chest to the hand. ( )
21. The three yang channels of the hand run from the hand to the head. ( )
22. The three yang channels of the foot run from the head to the foot. ( )
23. The three yin channels of the foot run from the foot to the head. ( )
24. Shangyang (LI 1) is often used in patients with: insomnia ( ), lumbar pain ( ), toothache ( ), sore and painful throat. ( )
25. According to the therapeutic principles of acupuncture one should reduce an

excess and tonify a deficiency. ( )

26. A patient should adopt a supine position when the point Huantiao (GB 30) is located. ( )

27. There are 27 points on the kidney channel. ( )

28. Points on the lung channel are indicated in cardiac, gastric and mental disorders. ( )

29. The distance between the transverse cubital crease and the transverse carpal crease is 16 cun. ( )

30. The course of the small intestine channel runs on the radial aspect of the little finger while the heart channel runs on the ulnar aspect. ( )

31. Neiguan (P 6) is indicated in disorders of the heart, stomach and chest. ( )

32. The point Sanyinjiao (Sp 6) is located at 3 cun directly above the tip of the external malleolus. ( )

33. Yin channels correspond to the Fu organs and connect with Zang organs while the Yang channels correspond to the Zang organs and connect with Fu organs. ( )

34. The eight confluent points in the extremities are where the twelve regular channels communicate with the eight extra channels. ( )

35. The Xi-Cleft points are used primarily to treat acute disorders. ( )

36. Renzhong (Renzhong) (Du 26) is indicated for toothaches. ( )

37. Zhongchong (P 9) is indicated for chiralgia. ( )

38. Gaohuang (B 43) is indicated for deficient syndromes.( )

39. Zhigou (SJ 6) is indicated for hypochondrium pain and constipation. ( )

40. Zhishi (UB 52) is indicated for impotence and involuntary emissions. ( )

41. Guilai (St 29) is indicated for disorders of the reproductive system. ( )

42. Utilizing the theory of the kidney dominating the bones, Taixi (K 3) can be used to treat toothaches. ( )

43. Deep insertion can not be applied to the point Gaohuangshu (UB 43). ( )

44. The needle should be inserted into the point Shuigou (Renzhong) (Du 26) to a depth of 0.5 cun when treating sudden loss of consciousness. ( )

45. The twelve regular channels all pass through or close to the throat, therefore all the regular channels, have points effective in treating sore throats. ( )

46. Utilizing the theory of "reinforcing the mother for deficiency syndrome while reducing the son for excess syndrome," Shaochong (H 9) and Yongquan (K 1) can be used to treat insomnia caused by a deficiency of heart yin.( )

47. Utilizing the theory of the "mother and son" relationship, when there is a liver excess (Shi) syndrome, the point Taichong (Liv 3) may be prescribed; in a

deficiency (Xu) syndrome, the point Zhongfeng (Liv 4) may be prescribed. (   )

Solutions to the Exercises

1. T, F, F, F, T; 2. F, T; 3. F; 4. F; 5. F; 6. T; 7. T; 8. F; 9. T; 10. F; 11. F; 12. F; 13. F; 14. F; 15. F; 16. F; 17. F; 18. T; 19. T; 20. T; 21. T; 22. T; 23. F; 24. F, F, F, T; 25. T; 26. F; 27. T; 28. F; 29. F; 30. F; 31. T; 32. F; 3 3. F; 34. F; 35. T; 36. F; 37. T; 38. T; 39. T; 40. T; 41. T; 42. T; 43. T; 44. T; 45. T; 46. F; 47. F.

III. Fill the Blanks

Example:

The three general functions of acu-points include <u>local therapeutic action</u>, <u>proximal therapeutic action</u> and <u>specific therapeutic action</u>.

1. The location for feeling the pulse is ________________ .

2. The three regions of Cun, Guan and Chi of the left hand reflect respectively the conditions of ____________ , ________ , and __________ ; and those of the right hand reflect conditions of ________ , ______ and ______ .

3. The Xi-Cleft points have the properties of treating ________ (acute or chronic) diseases occurring in their respective related organs. For example, __________ __________ of the stomach channel is effective for epigastric pain; __________ of the spleen channel of Foot-Taiyin is prescribed for menstrual pain.

4. ____________ , the Back-Shu point of the liver, may be chosen to treat ____ problems, as the ______ is the window of the liver; Shenshu (UB 23), the Back-Shu point of ______________ , can be selected to treat deafness, as the ear is the window of ____________ .

5. The five-Shu points are respectively attributed to the Five Elements. The order of the Five Elements in the yin channels is ________________________; the order in the yang channels is ____________________________ .

6. ____________ and __________ are two principles used to analyze and generalize the opposing forces of the anti-pathogenic and pathogenic factors during the course of a disease. Syndromes of the former one refer to ______________ ____ , the anti-pathogenic

factor is insufficient and the coordination of yin and yang impaired, while the influence of the path ogenic factor ________________________________. Syndromes of the latter one refer to those diseases in which the body function and the anti-pathogenic factor ________________________________, while the pathogenic factor __________ and severe struggle proceeds between ________________ and ____________________.

7. The theory of yin and yang mainly expounds ______________, ______________, ______________________________ and ________________________ relationship of yin and yang.

8. The theory of the Five Elements holds that ________, ________, ________, ______ and ______ are basic materials constituting the world.

9. The five categories of things classfied according to the Five Elements:

The Five Elements

	wood	*fire*	*earth*	*metal*	*water*
Zang organs	liver	heart	spleen	lung	
Fu organs		small intestine		large intestine	urinary bladder
Five sense organs	eye			nose	
Five tissues	tendon	vessel	muscle		
Emotions		joy		grief melancholy	fright fear

10. The theory of the Five Elements is applied to the medical field by using ________________, ________________, ____________ and ________________ relationships of the Five Elements to expound the interdepending and interrestraining relationships among the Zang-Fu organs, sense organs and tissues and also the relationship between man and nature.

11. The Five Elements are also used in ascertaining pathological conditions, for example, a greenish tinge in the complexion accompanied by preference for sour food suggests ________ disorders. Disorders of ________________ accompanid by a greenish complexion implies wood (liver) ________________ earth (spleen).

12. __________, ________, ________, ________, ________, and ________________ are known as the six Zang organs. Their main physiological functions

are production and storage of essential substance including ____________
____ , ____ , ________ and __________________ . The ______________
__ , __________________ , ________ , ______________ , ______________
____ , and ________ are known as the six Fu organs, their main funcitons being to ______________________ , ____________ and ________________ . There are also extra ordinary Fu organs, including ________ , ________ and uterus.

13. According to TCM, ____ , ________ and ____________ are fundamental substances in the human body for the maintenance of normal vital activities.

14. Both nutrient Qi (ying Qi) and defensive Qi (Wei Qi) are formed from __ ____________________________ . ________________ circulates in the vessels and supplies mainly the viscera. ______________ circulates outside the vessels and is mainly distributed in the muscles and skin to warm and nourish the subcutaneous tissues, and defend the body against exogenous pathogenic agents.

15. The nutrient essence derived from food through digestion and absorption by the __________ and __________ is transported to the ________ and ________ and transformed into red blood by the ____ and ____ .

16. Pathogenic factors are divided into the three groups: ________________ , ________________________ and ________________________________ .

17. The six exogenous pathogenic facotrs are ______ , ______ , __________ , ____ , ________ and ______ .

18. Among the seven emotional pathogenic factors, ________ injures the liver, __________________ injure the heart; ____________________ injure the lung; ____________ injures the spleen; and ____________ injures kidneys.

19. Clinically, disorders caused by the seven emotional pathogenic factors are seen mainly in the following three viscera: ____________ , ____________ and ________ .

20. Included in the category of miscellaneous pathogenic factors are ________ ______ , ______________________ or ________________________________ ________ , ________________ , ________________ and ______ .

21. ____________ , ________ and ____________ , ____________ , and ____ ____ are known as the four diagnostic methods in TCM.

22. The physiological functions of the channels and collaterals include ______ ____ .

23. Accidents during acupuncture treatment mainly include ______ , ________ ____ , ______________ , ______________ , _________ , and ___________________.

24. A patient complains of headache, blurring of the eye, hypochondriac distention, edema, constipation and ischuria, which can be diagnosed as disorder of the Sanjiao channel. If, according to the principle of matching of the Yuan and Luo points, the points ________ and ________ of the Sanjiao channel should be punctured; and according to the principle of matching of the Yuan and Luo points of the externally and internally related channels respectively, the Yuan point __ ________ of the Sanjiao channel and the Luo point ____________ of the pricardium channel should be punctured simultaneously.

25. The distance between Juque (Ren 14) and Shuifen (Ren 9) is __ cun.

26. The distance between Kunlun (UB 60) and Feiyang (UB 58) is __ cun.

27. The distance between Yinlingquan (SP 9) and Diji (SP 8) is __ cun.

28. The distance between Feiyang (UB 58) and Kunlun (UB 60) is __ cun.

29. The distance between Zhongshu (Du 7) and Shenzhu (Du 12) is __ cun.

30. The distance between Zhigou (SJ 6) and Sanyangluo (SJ 8) is __ cun.

31. The distance between the point Yindu (K 19) and Zhongwan (Ren 12) is __ cun.

32. The distance between the point Jingqu (Lu 8) and Kongzui (Lu 6) is __ cun.

33. The distance between the point Qiyangguan (GB 33) and Yanglinquan (GB 34) is __ cun.

34. The distance between Liangqiu (St 34) and Futu (LI 18) is __ cun.

35. The Back-Shu points of the five internal organs are ________ (UB 13), ____ ____ (UB 15), ________ (UB 18), ___________ (UB 20) and ___________ (UB 23). Their locations are: Feishu, ____ cun lateral to the lower border of the spinous process of the third thoracic vertebra; Xinshu, ____ cun lateral to the lower border of the spinous process of the fifth thoracic vertebra; Ganshu, ____ cun lateral to the lower border of the spinous process of the seventh thoracic vertebra; Pishu, ____ cun lateral to the lower border of the spinous process of the eleventh thoracic vertebra; Shenshu, ____ cun lateral to the lower border of the spinous process of the eleventh thoracic vertebra.

36. The distance between Chenfu (UB 36) and Yinmen (UB 37) is __ cun.

37. The distance between Shousanli (LI 10) and Fenglong (St 40) is __ cun.

38. The distance between Chize (Lu 5) and Kongzui (Lu 6) is __ cun.

39. The distance between Shousanli (LI 10) and Pianli (LI 6) is __ cun.

40. The proper order of moxibustion applied to the body is _________________ and/or the _______________ first and ___________________________ and/or ______ second; or ____ first, and ___________ second.

41. The auricular points are distributed on the auricle in a certain pattern. In general, the points located at ______ are related to the head and facial region, those on ________ to the upper limbs, those on ___________________________ to the trunk and lower limbs, and those in ___________________________ to the internal organs.

42. The eight extra confluent points are points in the extremitis connecting the eight extra channels and the twelve regular channels. Draw lines to link each of the following points with its belonging channels respectively.

Points	*Channels*
Gongsun (SP 4)	Yangwei
Neiguan (P 6)	Yinqiao
Houxi (SI 3)	Ren
Shenmai (UB 62)	Dai
Waiguan (SJ 5)	Yinwei
Zulinqi (UB 41)	Chong
Lieque (LU 7)	Du
Zhaohai (K 6)	Yangqiao

43. Tianshu (St 25) is located ______ lateral to the centre of the umbilicus. The point below the spinous process of the second lumbar vertebra is ______ .

44. ______ is 1.5 cun lateral to the lower border of the spinous process of the ninth thoracic vertebra. __________ (UB 67) is situated on the lateral side of the small toe, about (0.1 cun posterior to the corner of the nail.

45. Among the six Yang channels, ___________________ , ___________________ , _______________ and ___________________ are distributed to the centre of the auricle, and ________________________ to the periauricle.

46. The principles of matching of the acu-points include ___________________, _________________ and ____ .

47. The distance between the anterior and posteiror hairlines is taken as ____ cun, that between the transverse cubital crease and the transverse crease of the

wrist is __ cun, that between the sternocostal angle and the centre of the umbilicus is __ cun, and that between the prominence of the great trochanter and the middle of the patella is measured as __ cun.

48. Four of the eight confluent points are on the upper extremities, while the other four are on the lower extremities. The points on the upper extremities are frequently combined with those on the lower extremities. In the eight confluent points, for example, Neiguan (P 6) combined with Gongsun (Sp 4) is indicated in ______________________, _________________; Houxi (SI 3) combined with Shenmai (UB 62) is indicated in _________________, ___________, ________, and _____________; Waiguan (SJ 5) combined with Zulinqi (GB 41) is indicated in _____________________, ______, and _____________; and Lieque (Lu 7) and Zhaohai (K 6) in combination are indicated in _________________ ______, ________ and ____________.

49. The four different insertion methods of the filiform needle are ____, ______ __________, __________________________, and ________________________ __. The two manipulation methods of the needle include ____________ and __ ________.

50. In clinic, there are three most commonly used kinds of moxibustion, ______ ____________, _________________________, and _________________.

51. Clinically, four measuring methods have been established for locating acupoints on the body; they are _______________________________, ______ __________, ________________ and _________________.

52. __________ is located in the depression between the medial melleolus and tendo calcaneus, level with the tip of the medial malleolus. The point ________ ________ is at the tip of the middle finger.

53. The eight extraordinary channels are ______, ______, ______, ______, __ ____, ______, ______, and ________ channels.

54. According to the Xu-Shi (deficiency-excess) nature of the diseases, the manipulation methods of needles do not go beyond _______________, __________ __ and _________________.

55. The specific points include __________ points, ________ points, ______ points, ________ points, ________ point, ________ points, ______ points, __ __________ points, __________ points, and __________ points.

56. The main component of the channel-collateral system is the twelve regular channels. The order of circulation of Qi and blood in it is ____ → ____ → ____

→ ____ → ____ → ____ → ____ → ____ → ____ → ____ → ____ and in turn → ________________________ .

57. The eight confluent points are ________ , ________ , ________ , ________ , ________ , ________ , ________ and ________ .

Solutions to the Exercises

1. above the wrist where the radial artery throbs; 2. the heart, liver, kidney, the lung, spleen, kidney; 3. acute, Liangqiu (St 34), Diji (Sp 8); 4. Ganshu (UB 18), eye, eye, the kidney, the kidney; 5. wood → fire → earth → metal → water, metal → water → wood → fire → earth; 6. Deficiency, excess, those diseases in which the function of the human body is weak, has already become inconspicuous, is not to the point of impairment, is still of sufficient strength, is hyperactive, the antipathogenic, pathogenic factors; 7. the opposition, interdependence, interconsuming-supporting, inter-transforming; 8. wood, fire, metal, earth, water; 9. kidney, gall bladder, stomach, tongue, mouth, ear, skin and hair, bone, anger, meditation; 10. the interpromoting, interacting, overacting, counteracting; 11. liver, the spleen, overacting on; 12. The heart, liver, spleen, lung, kidney, pericardium, vi tal essence, Qi, blood, body fluid, small intestine, gallbladder, stomach, large intestine, urinary bladder, Sanjiao, recieve and digest food, transport, excrete wastes, the brain, uterus; 13. Qi, blood, body fluid; 14. essential substances in food, Nutrient Qi, Defensive Qi; 15. spleen, stomach, heart, lung, heart, lung; 16. the six exogenous factors, the seven emotional factors, miscellaneous pathogenic factors; 17. wind, cold, summer-heat, damp, dryness, heat; 18. anger, fright and excessive joy, grief and melancholy, meditation, fear; 19. heart, liver, spleen; 20. irrgegular food intake, overstrain and stress, lack of physical exertion, traumatic injuries, stagnant blood, phlegm; 21. inspection, auscultation, olfaction, inquiring, palpation; 22. promoting normal circulation of Qi and blood, connecting the superficial and interior portions of the human body and thus protecting it from attacks by etiological factors; 23. fainting, stuck needle, bent needle, broken needle, hematoma, after-effects; 24. Yangchi, Waiguan, Yangchi, Neiguan; 25. 5; 26. 7; 27. 3; 28. 7; 29. 7; 30. 1; 31. 0.5; 32. 6; 33. 3; 3 4. 4; 35. Feishu, Xinshu, Ganshu, Pishu, Shenshu, 1.5 cun, 1.5 cun, 1.5 cun, 1.5 cun, 1.5 cun; 36. 6; 37. 5; 38. 5; 39. 7; 40. the upper portion of the body, the back region, the lower portion of the body, the abdomen, head and trunk, the extremities; 41. the lobule, the scapha, the antihelix and its two crura, the cavum and cymba

conchae; 42.

Points	*Channels*
Gongsun (SP 4)	Yangwei
Neiguan (P 6)	Yinqiao
Nouxi (SI 3)	Ren
Shenmai (UB 62)	Dai
Waiguan (SJ 5)	Yinwei
Zulinqi (UB 41)	Chong
Lieque (LU 7)	Du
Zhaohai (K 6)	Yangqiao

43. 2 cun, Mingmen; 44. Ganshu, Zhiyin; 45. the large intestine channel, small intestine channel, Sanjiao channel, gallbaldder channel, the stomach and urinary bladder channels; 46. selection of local points, selection of proximal points, selection of points according to specific symptoms; 47. 12, 12, 8, 19; 48. diseases of the heart, chest and epigastric region, diseases of the neck, shoulder, back, inner canthus, diseases of the mastoid reigon, cheek, outer canthus, disorders of the throat, chest, lung; 49. inserting while pressuring, inseritng while fixing and pushing, inserting while stretching (the skin), inserting while pinching up (the skin), thrust-lifting, rotation; 50. with moxa cones, with moxa sticks, with warming needle; 51. according to anatomical landmarks, preportional measurement, finger measurement, simple measurement; 52. Taixi (K 3), Zhongchong (P 6); 53. Ren, Du, Chong, Dai, Yinwei, Yangwei, Yinqiao, Yangqiao; 54. reducing, reinforcing, even movement; 55. five-Shu, Yuan, Luo, Back-Shu, Front-Mu, Xi, eight confluent, crossing, lower He-Sea,eight influential; 56. the lung channel, large intestine channel, stomach channel, spleen channel, heart channel, small intestine channel, urinary channel, kidney channel, pericardium channel, gallbladder channel, liver channel, the lung channel; 57. Gongsun (Sp 4), Neiguan (P 6), Houxi (SI 3), Shenmai (UB 62), Zulinqi (GB 41), Waiguan (SJ 5), Lieque (Lu 7), Zhaohai (K 6).

IV. Definitions of TCM Terms

Try to explain the following TCM terms:

1. Differentiation of syndromes

This term refers to further analysis and synthesis of the clinical data obtained by the four diagnostic methods, to determine the stage to which a certain disease has developed, its location, and the degree of opposition between the body resistance and the pathogenic factors. In other words, identification is made not from a simple list of symptoms and signs but from a reflection of the pathogenes is of the disease.

2. The sea of all yang channels

The Du channel runs along the spinal column where all the yang channels meet, and so dominates the circulation of Qi and blood of these channels. The Du channel is thus called the sea of all yang channels.

3. The sea of all yin channels

The Ren channel is called the sea of all yin channels because the pathway of the channel runs along the middle of the chest and abdomen where all the yin channels meet.

4. Extraordinary points

These apply to those which have definite names and locations but are not listed in the system of the fourteen channels.

5. Ahshi points

These points are tender spots or sensitive spots present in certain diseases. They have neither definite locations nor names. In clinic, the tender spots or those with pathological changes usually determine the location of the Ahshi points.

6. Acupuncture sensation

When the needle is inserted with proper manipulation methods to a certain depth, the patient may feel soreness, numbness or distention around the points while the puncturist may experience a sensation of tightness and heaviness under the needle.

7. The theory of the Five Elements

It holds that wood, fire, earth, metal and water are basic materials constituting the material world. There exists among them an interdependence and inter-rest raint which determines their state of constant motion and change.

The theory of the Five Elements basically explains the interpromoting, interacting, over-acting and counter-acting relationship among them. Its applicaiton to TCM is in classifying into different categories natural phenomena plus the tissues and organs of the human body and the human emotions and interpreting the relationship between the physiology and pathology of the human body and the natural environment with the law of the inter-promoting, interacting, over-acting and counter-acting of the Five Elements. This theory is used as a guide in medical practice.

8. The over-acting relation of the Five Elements

It takes the form of launching an attack when a counterpart is weak. Clinically, this is conventionally called inter-acting. For example, wood over-acting on earth can also be called wood acting on earth. The order of over acting is the same as that of acting except that over-acting is not a normal inter-action but a harmful one occurring under certain conditions.

9. Zang-Fu organs

The term Zang-Fu in TCM refers to the gross anatomical entities of the internal organs. At the same time, it is also a generalization of the physiological functions of the human body. The heart, liver, spleen, lung, kidney and pericardium grouped together are known as the six Zang organs, their main physiological functions being to manufacture and store essential substances including vital essence , Qi, blood and body fluid. The small intestine, gallbladder, stomach, large intestine, urinary bladder and Sanjiao are known collectively as the Six Fu organs, whose main functions are to receive and digest food, absorb untrient substances , transmit and excrete wastes. There are in addition extraordinary Fu organs including the brain the the uterus.

10. The heart houses the mind

In TCM, the heart is considered the main organ governing mental activities and generalizing the physiological functions of the brain. Spirit, consciousness, memory, thinking and sleep are all dominated by these functions of the heart.

11. The liver opening into the eye

Each Zang-Fu organ has a certain influence on the functions of the eye. However, because the liver stores blood and its channel directly communicates with the eye, it has a closer relation to ocular functions, such as vision and movement of the eye, than other Zang-Fu organs.

12. The spleen dominates the muscles

Normal functioning of the spleen in transportation and transformation enables the muscles to receive adequate nourishment from the food essentials and thus maintains muscle thickness and strength.

13. The lung regulates water passages

The dispersing and descending functions of the lung regulate water passages and promote water metabolism. Its dispersing function turns a part of the body fluid into sweat to be excreted, while its descending function continuously sends a part of the body fluid down to the kidney and on to the urinary bladder to be excreted as urine.

14. The kidney receives Qi

Respiration is accomplished mainly by the lung, but the kidney helps through its function of controlling the reception of Qi. The distribution of the clean Qi inhaled by the lung to the whole body depends not only on the descending function of the lung but also on the kidney's function of reception and control.

15. Sanjiao and Lower Jiao

The channel of Sanjiao connects with the pericardium with which it is externally -internally related. Sanjiao is not a substantial organ, but a generalization of part of the functions of some of the Zang-Fu organs located in different sections of the body cavity.

Sanjiao is divided into three parts: Upper Jiao, Middle Jiao and Lower Jiao. Lower Jiao is a generalization of functions of the kidney and urinary bladder in controlling water metabolism as well as the storage and excretion of urine. It is like an aqueduct, a pathway for the flow of water.

16. Luo-Connecting points

Each of the twelve regular channels has a collacteral in the extremitis connecting a definite pair of yin and yang channels which are externally-internally related. In the trunk, there are the collaterals of the Ren and Du channels and the major collateral of the spleen distributed respectively in the posterior, anterior and lateral aspects of the body. Each of the collaterals has a Luo point, making 12 in all. A Luo point is used to treat diseases which involve the two externally-internally related channels and also diseases in the area supplied by the two channels.

17. The application of the Yuan-Source points and the Luo-Connecting points

The Yuan points are indicated in deficiency syndromes as well as excess syndromes of their respectively related organs. The Luo points of the twelve regular channels are indicated in the symptoms of their respective externally-internally related channels.

Clinically, these two groups of points can be used separately or coordinately. When a channel is affected, the Yuan point of that channel may be chosen as the main organ. The Luo point of the externally-internally related channel combines with the Yuan point to enhance the therapeutic effect.

V. Case Analysis

1. Patient A complains of dizziness and vertigo, accompanied by tinnitus,

flushed face, nausea, backache, redness of tongue proper and wiry and rapid pulse. Patient B also complains of dizziness and vertigo, but complications are fullness and suffocating sensation of the chest and epigastric reigon, profuse sputum, anorexia, a whitish sticky tongue coating, and a rolling pulse.

Differentiate the above two groups of symptoms presented by patient A and patient B, then prescribe for them respectively.

Key to the answer:
Symptoms presented by A can be categorized as upward attack of hyper-active yang of the liver. Application of reinforcing technique should be performed at the points Shenshu (UB 23) and Taixi (K 3) to strengthen kidney yin, and application of reducing technique at the points Ganshu (UB 18), Xingjian (Liv 2) and Fengchi (GB 20) to pacify yang of the liver. Symptoms presented by B can be diagnosed as interior retention of phlegm-damp. Reinforcing method should be applied to the points Pishu (UB 20) and Zhongwan (Ren 12) and reducing method should be applied to the points Fenglong (St-40) and Touwei (St 8). Taiyang (Extra) is an effective point for dizziness.

2. There are three types of vomitting described as follows. Read carefully the chief manifestations of each type to decide on the symptom-complex analysis, the manipulation method and the selection of the points.
A: Chief manifestations: Epigastric and abdominal distention or pain, acid fermented vomitus, belching, anorexia, constipation, and foul gas. The tongue is thickly coated and sticky, and the pulse is rolling and forceful.

Symptom-complex analysis: Retention of food.
Manipulation method: Reducing method.
Selection of points: Tianshu (St 25), Zusanli (St 36), Zhongwan (Ren 12), Neiguan (P 6) and Gongsun (Sp 4).

B: Chief manifestations: vomitting, acid regurgitation, continual belching, distending pain in the hypochondriac region, restlessness and irritability or depression. The tongue is thinly coated and sticky and the pulse wiry.

Symptom-complex analysis: Invasion of the stomach by Qi of the liver (or disharmony of the liver and stomach).

Manipulation method: Reducing method.
Selection of points: Taichong (Liv 3), Zusanli (St 36), Zhongwan (Ren 12), Neiguan (P 6) and Gongsun (Sp 4).

C: Chief manifestations: Sallow complexion, vomitting after eating a very full meal, lack of appetite, slightly loose stools, general lassitude, forceless pulse , thinly coated and sticky tongue.

Symptom-complex analysis: Deficiency of the spleen and stomach.
Manipulation method: Reinforcing method.
Selection of points: Pishu (UB 20), Zusanli (St 36), Zhongwan (Ren 12), Neiguan (P 6) and Gongsun (Sp 4).

3. A woman, aged 40, in May 1980 complained of a headache that had plagued her for many years. The history indicated bouts of right temporal pain that began 20 years ago, often preceded by nervous tension or overfatigue and aggravated furing menses. She experienced also boring pain in the right temporal region accompanied by cramping pain of the right eye. The bouts usually subsided after three days, sometimes with slight pain remaining. Modern examination showed no positive. Her case was diagnosed by the internist as one of vascular headache. Other positive findings obtaind with the traditional Chinese diagnostic procedures included: flushed face, restlessness, irritability, poor appetite with bitter taste in the mouth, constipation (one b.m. in two or three days), reddened tongue with a thin yellow coating, and a fin taut pulse, weak at the left cubit.

Questions:
Refer to the differentiation of syndromes according to the Zang-Fu organs and channels to decide whether the following diagnoses are true or false and explain.
A: This is a case of headache due to attack of wind on the Shaoyang channel.
B: This is a case of headache due to Shaoyang involvement, obstruction of liver Qi and exuberance of liver yang.
C: This is a case of headache caused by endogenous wind from the liver due to deficiency of yin and exuberance of liver yang.
(Key to the answer: A and B are false, C is true.)

It is wrong to attribute hemicrania to attack of channels by wind. When we speak of attack of channels by wind we are referring to attack by exogenous wind, which is characterized by paraxysmal pains and absence of any symptoms indicating involvement of internal viscera. Headache due to attack of channels by wind is an excessive symptom-complex which is not precipitated by fatigue or menses. On the other hand, this is a case of headache du to internal involvement that has nothing to do with exogenous wind.

Paraxysmal pains accompanied by synchronized eye involvement indicates the presence of wind, but rather than exogenous wind, it is endogenous wind from the liver du to deficiency of yin and exuberance of liver yang.

4. A woman aged 59 noted two months ago an increase in food intake and urinary output, accompanied by polydipsia, emaciation and lassitude. Signs of early cataract appeared soon after she was admitted into hospital with a diagnosis of diabetes, and her vision deteriorated. Funduscopic examination evealed hemorrhage on the left eye, with reading of 0.1 for the left eye and 0.01 for the right; symptoms suggesting diabetic involvement of the nervous system appearing at about the same time, including numbness of the digits and pain over the limbs distal to the elbows and knees. Examination also showed a reddish tongue with tooth prints but little coating, and a fine, weak and rapid pulse.

Questions:
1) Refer to the differentiation of syndromes according to the Zang-Fu organs and channels to decide whether the following diagnoses are true or false and explain.
A: This is a case of consumptive thirst (diabetes) with symptoms indicating pathological heat in the stomach.
B: This case can be diagnosed as consumptive thirst caused by deficiency of yin of the kidney and stomach.
C: This is a case of consumptive thirst due to blood stasis and obstruction of the channels.
D: A and B
E: B and C
F: A and C

(Answer: F)
(Key to the answer: Pathological heat in the stomach is indicated by numbness of the digits and pain over the limbs and failing vision resulting from deficiency of yin of the liver and obstruction of the liver channel).

2) According to the diagnosis made, which of the following prescriptions reflects completely the correct diagnosis and the principle of the treatment?

A: Taixi (K 3), Taichong (Liv 3), Shenshu (UB 23), Weiguan (SJ 5) and Jiaxi (St 41)
B: Taixi (K 3), Ganshu (UB 18), Zhongwan (Ren 12), Zusanli (St 36) and Sizhukong (SJ 23)
C: Rangu (K 2), Sanyinjiao (SP 6), Zhongwan (Ren 12), Zusanli (St 36), Waiguan (SJ 5) and Sizhukong (SJ 23)
(Key to the answer: Rangu, specific point for the treatment of diabetes, Sanyinjiao, Taixi, Taichong, Ganshu and Shenshu can be selected for replenishing the yin of

the liver and the kidney; Zusanli and Zhongwan, for regulating the functions of the stomach and spleen; and Sizhukong, Waiguan and Jiexi for invigorating the circulation of blood and the removal of blood stagnancy. In the light of the above analysis, one may find choice C is the right one including the essential acupoints to treat the disease).

3) What kind of manipulation should one use? (E)
A: Reinforcing technique
B: Reducing technique
C: Normal reinforcement and reduction
D: A and B
E: A,B and C
F: B and C
(Key to the answer: Reinforcing technique should be used at the points Rangu and Sanyinjiao; normal reinforcement and reduction used at the points Zhongwan, Zusanli, Waiguan and Sizhukong; reducing technique used at Sizhukong. The emaciation, lassitude, tooth prints and a fine, weak and rapid pulse all indicate deficiency of Qi. And reducing technique may harm the Qi further, while reinforcing technique would aggravate the heat in the stomach. That's why normal reducing and reinforcement are recommended. Cataract and fundic hemorrhage in this case are caused by exuberance of yang of the liver due to yin deficiency of the liver and the kidney, an indication to use reducing technique to depress the yang of the liver).

5. A woman aged 45 presented in November 1986 complained of "abnormal heart rhythm." As early as 1984 she was diagnosed as having rheumatic heart disease, mitral stenosis and moderate heart failure, and arrhythmia. Treatment with procaine amide and eraldin was started and continued both during her stay in hospital and after discharge one year later, but without definite improvement.

Findings on the four diagnostic methods all performed in the traditional way included palpitation, giddiness, exertional dyspnea, spontaneous sweating, lassitude, oliguria, diarrhea (3-6 b.m. per day), edema of the lower extremities, sensation of heat in the chest, preference for cold drinks, restlessness and dream-disturbed sleep, flushed cheeks, hot flashes in the face during menses, purple lips and purple swollen tongue with tooth prints, a watery tongue coating and a frequent, fine and deep pulse.

Questions:
1) Analyse the etiology presented by the patient (including determining which

viscera or bowels are involved and identifying with one or several of the eight principal syndromes).

Key to the answer:

The findings may be divided into four groups:
A: Deficiency of Qi of the heart indicated by palpitation, giddiness, exertional dyspnea, spontaneous sweating, lassitude, and deep pulse.
B: Deficiency of yin of the heart indicated by sensation of heat in the chest, preference for cold drinks, restlessness and dream-disturbed sleep, flushed cheeks, hot flashes in the face during menses and frequent and fine pulse.
C: Deficiency of Qi of the spleen indicated by oliguria, diarrhea and edema.
D: Blood stasis reflected by purple lips and tongue.

2) Try to decide on the line of treatment (including prescription and explanation).
Precription: Xinshu (UB 15), Jueyinshu (GB 14), Juque (Ren 14), Shanzhong (Ren 1 7), Geshu (UB 17), Neiguan (P 6), Shenmen (H 7), Diji (Sp 8), Zhaohai (K 6) and Zusanli (St 36)

Use reinforcing method and retain the needles for 30 minues each time. Treat once a day, with ten days to a course. Rest 2-3 days between courses.

Explanation:

Jueyinshu and Shanzhong, the front and back points of the pericardium, are selected because the pericardium is often involved first and the heart is subsequently invaded by exogenous evil factors. Shanzhong is chosen also because it is the strategic point of Qi. Since this is a case of blood stasis, so Geshu, the strategic point of blood, is chosen to activate blood circulation and relieve blood stasis. However, as Qi is the commander of blood, promoting the normal flow of Qi is prerequisite to activating blood circulation, a situation indicating the use of Shanzhong. Diji is the point of choice because this point, the cleft point of the spleen channel, helps relieve edema, abdominal distention and dyspnea. Zhaohai, one of the eight confluent points of the kidney channel, connects with the heart via the lung, so besides antipyretic and tranquilizing aciton, acupuncture of Zhaohai helps relieve edema. Neiguan is both the connecting point of the pericardium channel of Hand-Jueyin, and a point of the regulating channel of yin. It is always reasonable to consider Neiguan as a primary choice in dealing with heart problems. Zusanli is selected to invigorate the Qi of the spleen. Shenmen, the Yuan point of the heart channel, may calm the heart and soothe the mind. Xinshu and Juque, the Back-Shu and Front-Mu points of the heart, have the properties of regulating Qi and blood of the heart and as a tranquilizer.

6. Differentiate the syndromes of irregular menstruation according to the different clinical manifestations presented below and then form a proper prescription for each of them.

1) Menstruation with shortened cycle, profuse, dark-purple and sticky menstrual flow accompanied by thirst, restlessness, a red tongue with a yellow coating.

Diagnosis and differentiation of syndromes: Menstruation with shortened cycle caused by heat of blood resulting in hemorrhage.

Prescription: Zhongji (Ren 3), Sanyinjiao (Sp 6), Taichong (Liv 3) and Xuehai (S p 10).

Needling by reducing method should be applied so as to exert and action of clearing up the heat and cooling the blood.

2) Menstruation with shortened cycle, profuse, thin and light-coloured menstruous flow accompanied by pallor, lassitude, a pale tongue coating and a weak pulse.

Diagnosis and differentiation of syndromes: Menstruation with shortened cycle due to deficiency of Qi failing to control the blood circulation.

Prescription: Qihai (Ren 6), Diji (SP 8) and Zusanli (St 36). Needling by reinforcing method should be applied in order to tonify the Qi to control the blood.

3) Menstruation with prolonged cycle, scanty and dark-reddish menstrual flow, accompanied by lower abdominal pain alleviated by hot compress, aversion to cold, chillness of the extremities, pallor, a pale tongue with a scanty, whitish coating and a deep-tightish pulse.

Diagnosis and differentiation of syndromes: Menstruation with prolonged cycle caused by blood-cold.

Prescription: Moxibustion should be applied to the points Zhongji (Ren 3), Sanyinjiao (Sp 6), Mingmen (Du 4) and Guanyuan (Ren 4) so as to warm the yang and disperse the cold.

4) Menstruation with prolonged cycle: scanty and light-coloured menstrual flow accompanid by a sallowish face, palpitation, a pale tongue with scanty coating, and a weak, thready pulse.

Diagnosis and differentiation of syndromes: Menstruation with prolonged cycle caused by blood deficiency.

Prescription: Reinforcing method should be applied when puncturing the points Xinshu (UB 15), Geshu (UB 17) and Pishu (UB 20) in order to tonify the spleen to produce blood.

5) Menstruation with prolonged cycle: scanty and dark-coloured menstrual flow accompanied by lower abdominal distention and pain, stuffiness in the chest, tenderness of breasts, hypochondriac pain, a dark-red tongue and a wiry pulse.

Diagnosis and differentiation of syndromes: Menstruation with prolonged cycle caused by stagnation of liver Qi.

Prescription: Reducing method should be performed on the points Zhongji (Ren 3), Neiguan (P 6), Zhongwan (Ren 12) and Xingjian (Liv 2) to remove stagnation of liver Qi.

7. Mr. Zhang, aged 50, on December 3, 1986 complained of swelling and pain of the knee joints for the past half month. The pain considerably disturbed the movements of the affected knee joints, but it seemed to be alleviated only when hot compress was applied. Examination showed no discolour but swelling on the affected area. The tongue coating was white and the pulse was deep-tight.

Diagnosis and differentiation of syndromes: Bi (obstruction) syndrome caused by invasion of exogenous cold, resulting in stagnation of the Qi and blood in the channels and collaterals.

Prescription: Dubi (St 35), Yanglingquan (GB 34), Liangqiu (St 34), Qiyangguan (GB 33), Shenshu (UB 23) and Guanyuan (Ren 4)

Manipulation method: Acupuncture by even movement for 30 minutes, together with moxibustion.

8. Differentiate the syndromes of the following cases, make a clear diagnosis reflecting perspectives of TCM and form a prescription for each of them.

1) Mr. Wan, aged 51, complained of soreness in the loins and knees. Other symptoms included dizziness, tinnitus and insomnia. Examination showed a red tongue and a deep, thready pulse.

Diagnosis and differentiation of syndromes: Insomnia caused by deficiency of kidney yin.

Prescription: Shenmen (H 7), Sanyinjiao (Sp 6), Shenshu (UB 23), Taixi (K 3) and Anmian (Extra).

2) Ms. Zhan, aged 48, complained of headache, vertigo, irascibility and bitter taste in the mouth after she had quarrelled with her colleague three days before. Examination showed a red tongue with a thin, yellowish coating, and a forceful, wiry pulse.

Diagnosis and differentiation of syndromes: Headache caused by depression of liver Qi which has turned into flare-up of liver fire.

Prescription: Fengchi (GB 20), Baihui (Du 20), Taiyang (Extra 2), Xingjian (Liv 2) and Jiaxi (GB 43).

3) Miss Song, aged 21, of a weak constitution, suffered from abdominal pain after menstruation accompanied by scanty flow, poor appetite, soreness in the loins and knees, a pale tongue with a whitish coating, and a weak and deep pulse.

Diagnosis and differentiation of syndromes: Dysmenorrhea due to deficiency of Qi and blood.

Prescription: Mingmen (Du 4), Shenshu (UB 23), Zusanli (St 36) and Guanyuan (Ren 4) (acupuncture by reinforcing method together with moxibustion).

4) Mr. Wang, aged 38, in the past three years had suffered from epigastric pain which seemed to have worsened recently. The pain usually started two hours after meal, radiating to the back and hypochondria and lasting a long period of time. Other symptoms accompanied were nausea, vomiting sour and bitter fluid, belching, poor appetite, abdominal distention, a thin, whitish tongue coating and a deep , wiry pulse.

Diagnosis and differentiation of syndromes: Epigastric pain caused by stagnation of liver Qi causing failure of the Qi of the stomach to descend.

Prescription: Points mainly on the liver and stomach channels
Zhongwan (Ren 12), the Front-Mu point of the stomach channel.
Zusanli (St 36), the He-Sea point of the stomach channel.
Taichong (Liv 3), the Yuan point of the liver channel.
Qimen (Liv 14), the Front-Mu point of the liver channel.

9. Make a prescription for each of the following cases by basing on the therapeutic principle that you will decide on first.

1) Ms. Xiao, aged 34, had a history of asthma for five years. The condition had become worse in the past two days because of cold weather. Other positives were headache, painful joints, chillness, cough, chest, pain and insomnia. Examination showed a whitish tongue coating and a floating, slippery pulse.

Therapeutic principle: Disperse exterior pathogenic cold and tonify the lung so as to strengthen the defensive ability of the body surface.

Prescription: Fengchi (GB 20), Waiguan (SJ 5) and Lieque (Lu 7) should be punctured in combination with moxibustion on the points Zusanli (St 36), Feishu

(UB 13) and Tianshu (St 25).

2) Mrs. Liu, aged 37, complained of sharp paroxysmal pain in the lower abdomen two days before or during the menstruation. The accompanying symptoms were headache and dizziness. Examination showed a thin, whitish tongue coating and a wiry pulse. All of the symptoms seemed to be gone after the mense.

Therapeutic principle: Activate the Qi of the liver and promote the circulation of blood.

Prescription: Zhongji (Ren 3), Uterus (Extra), Hegu (LI 4), Sanyinjiao (Sp 6) and Xingjian (Liv 2).

3) Yi, male, aged 5, had a high-grade fever half a month before. After receiving 3-day drug treatment, the temperature reduced considerably but the limbs remained so weak that the right hand failed to raise and the right leg failed to walk normally.

Therapeutic principle: Regulate the Qi in the channels and collaterals.

Prescription: Jianyu (LI 15), Jianliao (SJ 14), Quchi (LI 11), Hegu (LI 4) and Jiaji (Extra) points on the upper chest. Huantiao (GB 30), Liangqiu (St 34), Yanglingquan (GB 34), Zusanli (St 36), Kunlun (UB 60) and Jiaji (Extra) points in the lumbar region.

4) Ms. Yu, aged 38, complained of having sudden stiffness sensation in the ears the previous night. The condition became worse in the morning accompanied by tinnitus, dizziness a thin, yellowish tongue coating and a wiry pulse.

Therapeutic principle: Subdue the endogenous wind caused by hyperactivity of the liver so as to benefit the ear.

Prescription: Fengchi (GB 20), Taichong (Liv 3), Ermen (SJ 21) and Yifeng (SJ 17).

5) Ms. Chen, aged 41, complained of epigastric distention and pain radiating to the hypochondriac region, nausea and insomnia. Examination showed a thin, yellowish tongue coating and a wiry pulse.

Doctor A wanted to use the points Zhongwan (Ren 12), Neiguan (P 6), Zusanli (St 36) and Taichong (Liv 3), and doctor B wanted to use the points Liangmen (St 21), Neiguan (P 6), Zusanli (St 36) and Neiting (St 44).

Question: Which of the two doctors is right in selecting the points and why? If neither of them is right, write out your prescription and explanation.

Answer: Doctor A is right though two of the points suggested by Doctor B are also proposed by Doctor A.

Explanation: As the patient's epigastric distention and pain radiates to the hypochondriac region, it can be classified under the category of invasion of liver Qi on the stomach. Other symptoms such as nausea, insomnia, thin yellowish tongue coating and wiry pulse also indicate a syndrome of obstructed liver Qi leading to fire. The therapeutic principle, therefore, should be focused on removing the stasis of liver Qi, clearing up the fire as well as regulating the function of the affected stomach so as to relieve pain. The points selected accordingly should be Zhongwan, Zusanli and Neiguan for relieving pain and Taichong for renormalizing the function of the liver. Besides, it would be better if the point Xingjian is employed to complement Taichong.

10. Ms. Bi aged 38, complained of frequent pain on the forehead which usually became worse in the afternoon. Other symptoms were palpitation, restlessness, dizziness, anorxia, red tongue and thready pulse.

Diagnosis: headache (due to deficiency of blood).

Therapeutic principle: Nourish yin and tonify blood and activate circulation of the channel in the head.

Prescription: Yintang (Extra 1), Hegu (LI 4), Sanyinjiao (Sp 8), Geshu (UB 17) and Taixi (K 3).

Explanation: Pain in the forehead belongs to disorder of the stomach channel of Foot-Yangming, so the point Yintang of the stomach channel, and the remote point Hegu are selected to activate circulation of Qi in the head region. The points Sanyinjiao, Geshu and Taixi are used for the purpose of tonifying blood and housing the mind. In addition, the point Zusanli can also the punctured considering the patient's poor appetite.

VI. Questions and Answers

1. What is acupoint?

Answer: An acupoint is a stimulated region in acupuncture and moxibustion. It is the place on the body surface where the Qi of the channels and collaterals and Zang-Fu organs infuse and pool and so is also called a point of Qi.

2. What are the eight principles in differentiation of syndromes and which are the chief principles among them and why?

Answer: The eight principles are exterior and interior, cold and heat, Xu (defi ciency) and Shi (excess) and yin and yang. Yin and yang are the chief principles among the eight as the exterior, heat and Shi syndromes can all be classified as yang, while the interior cold and Xu syndromes can all be categorized as of the yin type.

3. What is the channel phenomenon?

Answer: Channel phenomenon refers to the phenomenon of a propagated sensation along the channels. It implies the phenomenon of propagation of a specific sensation along the pathways of classical channels on the human body when the points are stimulated.

4. What are specific points?

Answer: Among the points of the fourteen channels, those which have specific properties are called specific points. They are grouped together under special names, such as Five-Shu points, Yuan-Source points, Luo-Connecting points, Xi-Cleft points, Back-Shu points, Front-Mu points, eight crossing points, eight confluent points and lower He-Sea points.

5. What is the principle of matching of Shu-Mu and Yuan-Luo points? Give an example to show its application to acupuncture clinics.

Answer: The Back-Shu points and the Front-Mu points are used more in combination than used alone. Whenever an organ is affected, the Back-Shu points and the Front-Mu points of the same organ can be prescribed. For example, Weishu on the back and Zhongwan on the abdomen may be selected for gastric disorders. Clinically, the combination of the Yuan and Luo points is conventionally used when a channel is affected; the Yuan points of the channel may be chosen as radical points, while the luo points on its externally-internally related channel combined with it to enhance the therapeutic results. The most commonly seen matching of Yuan and Luo points is that the point Taiyuan (Lu 9), the Yuan point of the lung channel , and the point Pianli (LI 6), the Luo point of the large intestine channel, are prescribed if the lung channel is affected.

6. State briefly what the proper way is of doing manipulation in terms of reinforcement, reduction as well as normal reinforcement and reduction.

Answer: Key points: Lifting, thrusting, twisting and rotating the needle are the most commonly used methods for reinforcement and reduction. Reinforcement consists in first doing shallow insertion before going deeper; thrusting the needle rapidly with force while lifting it slowly with little force; small depth deference between thrusting and lifting and low frequency of movements; slow twisting and rotating with little force and in small amplitude. Reduction is just the opposite.

As for normal reinforcement and reduction, all these movements are doen evenly with moderate speed and force.

7. What is the basic principle of adopting proper posture of the patient during acupuncture treatment? What specific posture should the patient use while receiving acupuncture at the points Tiantu (Ren 22), Dubi (St 35), Dazhui (Du 14) and Zhongwan (Ren 12)?

Answer: Full exposure of the points selected to be punctured determines the patient's position during acupuncture treatment. The acupuncturist must be able to perform without hindrance, while the patient must relax himself and make himself comfortable. For example, the patient should use a recumbent position for the puncturing of the Dubi point, a sitting, slightly bending position for the puncturing of the Dazhui point, and a supine position for the puncturing of the Zhongwan point.

8. How is the substantial phlegm to be distinguished from the nonsubstantial phlegm?

Answer: In the etiology of TCM, phlegm involves the following two aspects: Substantial phlegm: This may refer to pathological products, e.g. sputum. They are secondary pathological factors which will lead to further pathological changes if not eliminated in time. Non-substantial phlegm: This is sometimes a pathological concept generalizing the characteristics of the clinical symptoms and signs. For example, a case of epilepsy with coma and rattle in the throat can be diagnosed from the characteristics of the clinical manifestation as "the heart being misted by the phlegm."

9. What are the meanings of Sanjiao, upper Jiao, middle Jiao and lower Jiao?

Answer: Sanjiao is not a substantial but an isolated organ. It is a generalization of part of the functions of some of the Zang-Fu organs located in different selections of the body cavity. Sanjiao is divided into three parts:

1) Upper Jiao is a generalization of the function of the heart and lung in transporting Qi and blood to nourish various parts of the body. It is like an all-pervading vapour.

2) Middle Jiao is a generalization of the function of the spleen and stomach in digestion and absorption. This may be compared to soaking things in water to cause decomposition and dissolution of substances.

3) Lower Jiao is a generalization of functions of the kidney and urinary bladder in controlling water metabolism as well as storage and excretion of urine. It is

like an aqueduct, a pathway for the flow of water.

10. What are the four kinds of relationships among the Five Elements? Among the four, which one(s) can be categorized as physiological phenomenon(a), and which one(s) otherwise?

Answer: The four kinds of relationships are the inter-promoting, interacting, over-acting and counter-acting relationships. The former two can be categorized as physiological phenomena, but the latter two as pathological phenomena.

11. What are the meanings of over-acting and counter-acting? What are their proper orders in the Five Elements?

Answer: Over-acting means launching an attack when a counterpart is weak. Clinically, this is conventionally called inter-acting. In the Five Elements, the order is that wood over-acts on earth, earth on water, water on fire, fire on metal, and metal on earth.

Counter-acting denotes prey upon (other elements). The order is just opposite to that of over-acting.

12. Fill in the blanks with proper words by using the Five Elements theory.

Answer: [fire] $\xleftarrow{\text{Counter-acting}}$ metal (in excess) $\xrightarrow{\text{over-acting}}$ [wood]

[fire] $\xrightarrow{\text{over-acting}}$ metal (in deficiency) $\xleftarrow{\text{Counter-acting}}$ [wood]

Explanation: The phenomena of over-acting and counter-acting caused by excess or deficiency of any one of the Five Elements often manifest themselves simultaneously. In the Figure shown above, when metal is in excess it not only over-acts on wood, but also counter-acts on fire; when metal is in dieficiency, it is over- acted on by fire and counter-acted on by earth at the same time.

13. What are the five-Shu points? What are the principles of mother-invigoration and child-purgation in selection of points?

Answer: The five-Shu points, Jing-Well, Ying-Spring, Shu-Stream, Jing-River and He-Sea, are five specific acupoints of the twelve channels situated below the elbows and knees and along which the vital energy of the channels flows.

Mother-invigoration and child-purgation imply needling the five-Shu points according to the law of generation and restriction of the Five Elements theory. When an organ or channel is asthenic, therefore, needle the mother-point of the same channel or that of its mother channel; in asthenia syndrome, needled the child-point of the same channel or that of its child channel. In asthenia syndrome of the liver, for example, the indication is to needle either the water point of the liver channel, Ququan (Liv 8), which is the mother point of the same channel, or the water point of the kidney channel, Yingu (K 10), which is the mother-point of the mother channel. In asthenia syndromes of the liver, one of the five- Shu points of the same channel, Xingjian (Liv 2), which is the child-point of the same channel, or that of the child-channel (the heart), Shaofu (H 8), is indicated.

14. What does "arrival of Qi" mean?

Answer: When the needle is inserted to a certain depth, the patient may feel soreness, numbness or distention around the point. The operator at the same time may feel tenseness around the needle. This is called "arrival of Qi," indicating the needling has produced its effect in calling the channels and collaterals into function.

15. What would you do if Qi is absent after the reinforcing or reducing procedure is applied?

Answer: In that case, the operator should check to see whether the point is located accurately or the direction of the needle is correct. If Qi still does not arrive, the needle may be retained for a short time, or manipulated gently with lift-thrust movements. The needle reaction may also be induced by such auxiliary manipulaitons as:

1) Twirling the needle: Do it with the thumb and index finger of the right hand in one direction with an amplitude of 360° or more, repeatng the manipulation once or twice if necessary.

2) Scraping of the handle of the needle: When the needle is retained, steady it by placing the thumb of the right hand lightly on top of it, then scrape the handle with the nail of the index or middle finger upward from the bottom.

3) Vibrating the needle: Hold the needle with the right hand and apply quick lift-thrust movement with small amplitude to cause vibration. Delay in the arrival of Qi in some patients may be due to local obstruction of the channels. In that case, cease forceful manipulation and apply mild moxibustion, or selected other points to evoke the vital energy of the channels. There are patients, however, with weak constitution who find no response to needling by whatever method. For these patients no therapeutic results can be expected.

16. What is the relationship between the five-Shu points and the Five Elements?

Answer: On yang channels: Well—metal, Xing—water, Shu—wood, Jing—fire, He—earth.

On yin channels: Well—wood, Xing—fire, Shu—earth, Jing—metal, He—water.

17. Try to write out two main indications of each of the following acupoints.

Answer:

1) Gongsun (Sp 4)—stomachache and abdominal pain
2) Quchi (LI 11)—cardiac pain and pain in the elbow
3) Taichong (Liv 3)—headache and convulsion
4) Guangming (GB 37)—eye disorders and pain in the lower extremities
5) Shengshu (UB 23)—lumbar pain and involuntary emission
6) Jiache (St 6)—facial paralysis and toothache
7) Tiantu (Ren 22)—asthma and sore throat
8) Taiyang (Extra 2)—headache and eye problem
9) Zhigou (SJ 6)—hypochondriac pain and constipation
10) Zusanli(St 36) Stomach ache and pain in knee joints

18. Write out six local points that can be used in treating painful ankle.
Answer: Shenmai (UB 62), Zhaohai (K 6), Kunlun (UB 60), Qiuxu (GB 40), Shangqiu (SP 5) and Jiexi (St 41)

19. What are the main indications of the following acupoints? Huantiao (GB 30), Dazhui (Du 14), Waiguan (SJ 5) and Xuanzhong (GB 39)
Answer:
Huantiao—sciatic neuralagia, lumbago and leg pain
Dazhui—fever, common cold, asthma, cough and stiff neck
Waiguan—common cold, pneumonia, deafness and migraine
Xuanzhong—pain in the knee, ankel and lower chest, hemiplegia, and sciatic neuralgia

20. What are the main clinical manifestations of dysmenorrhea due to deficiency syndrome? What are the commonly used prescription and manipulation?
Answer: The main manifestations are lower abdominal pain at the late stage of, or after, menstruation, mild but persistent pain responding to warmth and pressure, menstruation, mild but persistent pain responding to warmth and pressure, menstrual flow scanty and pinkish in colour.
Prescription: Acupuncture with reinforcing method together with moxibustion are applid to Guanyuan (Ren 4), Pishu (UB 20), Shenshu (UB 23), Zusanli (St 36) and Sanyinjiao (Sp 6).

21. Which channels distribute to the auricle area?
Answer:
1) The small intestine channel of Hand-Taiyang.
2) The large intestine channel of Hand-Yangming.
3) The urinary bladder channel of foot-Taiyang.

4) The gallbladder channel of Food-Shaoyang.
5) The Sanjiao channel of Hand-Shaoyang.

22. How to puncture the point Tianshu (St 25) correctly?

Answer: First puncture 0.2-0.3 cun obliquely and then puncture about 1.5 cun horizontally with the needle point directed downward along the posterior surface of the manubrium.

23. What are the commonly used methods of matching acupoints?

Answer:

1) Matching of points on the back and on the front region, i.e. matching of the Shu-Mu points.
2) Matching of points on the lower and upper portions, i.e. matching of the eight confluent points.
3) Matching of the points on the left and right of the body, i.e. selecting points of the left side to treat disease of the right side, and vice versa.
4) Matching of the local and remote points, i.e. matching of Hegu and Dicang points for the treatment of facial paralysis.
5) Matching of the points on externally-internally related channels, i.e. matching of the points Hegu and Yuji for the treatment of sore throat.

24. What are the commonly used reinforcing and reducing methods?

Answer: Some of the frequently used methods include:

(a) Lifting and thrusting the needle: The effect of reinforcing and reducing is achived through the speed and the force in repeated lifting and thrusting of the needle. In reinforcing, once the needling sensation is felt, lift the needle gently and slowly, then thrust in heavily and rapidly. In reducing, lift the nedle forcefully and rapidly, then thrust gently and slowly.

(b) Method of rotating the needle: The effect of reinforcing and reducing depends on the amplitude and speed of the needle rotation. In reinforcing, when the needle reaches a certain depth, rotate it back and forth continuously with small amplitude and slowly. In reducing, rotate the needle continuously back and forth with large amplitude and rapidly.

(c) Even movement: This method is used in treating diseases typical of both the Xu and Shi nature. Application is by inserting the needle to a certain depth till sensation is felt, and at moderate speed to cause a mild sensation. The needle is withdrawn also at moderate speed.

25. What is the purpose of needle-retention?

Answer: After the needle is inserted into a point, it should be retaind in position for from several minutes to hours depending on the individual pathological condition. This is for the purpose of (1) strengthening the acupuncture sensation, especially in treating patients with chronic, painful or spasm disorders; (2) making patients feel acupuncture sensation, espcially those who are not responsive to acupuncture.

26. Mark out the auricular points.

Answer: Sympathetic, adrenal gland, subcortex, endocrine, occiput, Shenmen, brain stem and liver in Fig. 10 (based on Chinese auricular chart).

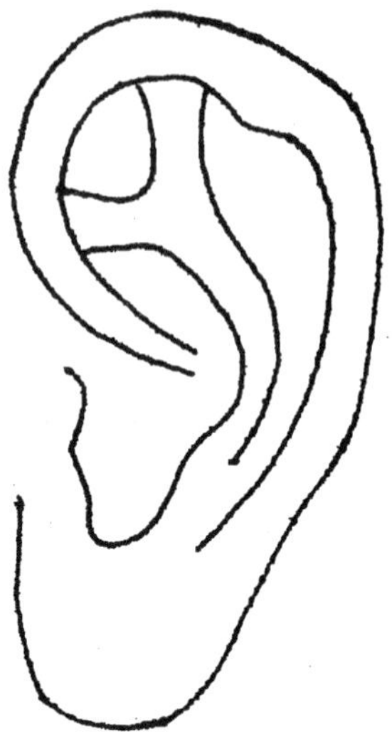

Fig. 10

27. What are the functions of moxibustion?

Answer: Moxibustion has the properties of warming and removing obstacles of the channels, eliminating cold and damp, so it is used in treatment of dizziness, anemia, galactozemia, amenorrhea caused by invasion of wind, cold and damp, or deficiency of Qi and blood. Moxibustion also has the function of treating diseases such as chronic diarrhea or dysentry, enuresis, urine bleeding, prolapse of the rectum, etc. Moxibustion used as a subsidiary means is effective in treating mastitis and furuncle in their early stage. In addition, moxibustion on the points Dazhui (Du 14), Guanyuan (Ren 4), Qihai (Ren 6) and Zusanli (St 36) is usually performed for a preventive and health-care purpose as it can promote the defensive Qi of the body surface to strengthen the resistance.

28. What are the main factors causing fainting during acupuncture treatment and what is the commonly seen symptoms indicating fainting? How to manage it?

Answer: Fainting may occur due to weakness or to nervous tension on receiving acupuncture for the first time, or to too forceful manipulation. The prodromes are dizziness and vertigo, irritability, nausea, pallor, staring eyes and dull appearance. In severe cases, there may be shock and unconsiousness, and deep pulse. Th e needles should be removed at once and the patient asked to relax and the operator should help her/him to lie down. In mild cases, offer the patient warm drinks. The symptoms will disappear after a short rest. In severe cases, press Renzhong (Du 26) with the fingernails or puncture Renzhong (Ren 26) and

Zhongchong (P 9). Moxibustion may be applied to Baihui (Du 20) and Zusanli (St 36). Generally the patient will respond, but if not, then other emergency measures should be taken.

29. What are the functions of channels and collaterals?

Answer: The functions of channels and collaterals consist of circulating Qi and blood, warming and nourishing the tissues and linking up the whole body so as to keep the Zang-Fu organs, four limbs, skin, muscles, tendons and bones intact in structure and functioning synergically and make the body an organic integrity. These functions of the channels and collaterals play an important role in clinical work. In acupuncture and moxibustion therapy the affected channels or Zang-Fu organs are first detected. Points are then selected from adjacent areas or from the corresponding channels in distant areas. Therapeutic results may be obtained through regulating the circulation of the Qi and blood in the channels and collaterals.

30. How do you prescribe in treating headache according to its locality and its supplying channels?

Answer: Pain at the forehead and supraorbital region being related to the stomach channel of Foot-Yangming, the points Yintang (Extra), Zuanzhu (UB 2), Hegu (LI 4) and Neiting should be selected. Pain at the occipital region and nape being related to the urinary bladder channel of Foot-Taiyang, and points Fengfu (Du 16), Tianzhu (UB 10) and Jinmen (GB 25) may be used. Pain at the temporal region of both sides or only one side being related to the gallbladder channel of Foot-Shaoyang, the points Taiyang (Extra 2), Xuanlu (GB 5), Waiguan (SJ 5) and Zulinqi (GB 41) should be punctured. The points Baihui (Du 20), Taichong (Liv 3) and Yongquan (K 1) should be employed for pain at the parietal region which is related to the liver channel of Foot-Jueyin.

31. What does the statement "Where a channel traverses, there the place is amenable to treatment" mean?

Answer: It is an old saying meaning selection of points according to the distribution of the channels, that is, select points the channel of which traverses the site of the operation.

32. What are the names and meanings of the eight confluent points?

Answer: The eight confluent points are points in the extremities connecting the eight extra channels and the twelve regular channels. These points have the therapeutic effect on treating diseases of the extra channels and their related regular channels. Four of these eight points, namely, Neiguan, Houxi, Waiguan and

Lieque, are on the upper extremities, while the other four, namely Gongsun, Shenmai, Zulinqi and Zhaohai, are on the lower extremities.

33. What are the six lower He-Sea points of the Fu organs? What are their functions?

Answer: The lower He-Sea points of the Fu organs usually give satisfactory results in treating diseases of the six Fu organs, the reason being that the Fu organs are closely related to the three yang channels of the foot, and each has a lower He-Sea point. They are Zusanli, the lower He-Sea point of the stomach channel; Shangjuxu, the lower He-Sea point of the large intestine; Xiajuxu, the lower He-Sea point of the small intestine channel; Yanglingquan, the lower He-Sea point of the gallbladder channel; Weizhong, the lower He-Sea point of the urinary bladder channel; and Weiyang, the lower He-Sea point of the Sanjiao channel. At the same time, the three yang channels of the foot ocmmunicate with the three yang channels of the hand. In treating diseases of the six Fu organs, the main points selected are the lower He-Sea points.

34. Write out the locations and indications of the acupoints Fengchi (GB 20), Zhaohai (K 6), Ganshu (UB 18) and Tinghui (GB 2).

35. How many types of apoplexy are classified according to the degree of severity? Prescribe for each type.

Answer: In general, there are two types of windstroke according to the degree of severity: the severe type or what is called the Zang-Fu organs being attacked showing symptoms and signs of the channels and collaterals and the viscerae; the mild type or what is conventionally called the channels and collaterals being at tacked, the symptoms and signs pertaining to the channels and collaterals. In treating hemiplegia of the mild type, the points Jianyu (LI 15), Quchi (LI 11), Waiguan (SJ 5), Hegu (LI 4), Huantiao (GB 20), Yanglingquan (GB 34), Zusanli (St 36) and Juegu (GB 39) are selected; in treating facial paralysis of this type, Dicang (St 4), Jiache (St 6), Neiting (St 44) and Taichong (Liv 3) are punctured on the diseased side in the early stage and on both sides in the later stage. For the tense syndrome of the severe type, Shuigou (Du 26), Taichong (Liv 3), Fenglong (St 40) and Laogong (P 8) and the twelve Jing points are punctured by reducing method with filiform needles or with a three-edged needle to cause slight blood; and for the flaccid syndrome of the severe type, continuous indirect moxibustion with salt may be applied to the points Guanyuan (Ren 4), Shenque (Ren 8) and Qihai (Ren 6).

36. Describe the locations and indications of the points on the toe.

Answer:

1) Yinbai (Sp 1)
Location: on the medial aspct of the hallux, about 0.1 cun proximal to the corner of the toenail.
Indications: Abdominal distention, menometrorrhagia, etc.
2) Dadun (Liv 1)
Location: on the lateral aspect of the dorsum of the hallux, 0.1 cun proximal to the corner of the toenail.
Indications: Prolapse of the uterus, painful hernia, etc.
3) Lidui (St 45)
Location: on the lateral side of the 2nd toe, about 0.1 cun posterior to the corner of the toenail.
Indications: Facial swelling, deviation of the mouth, toothache, febrile diseases, cold in the leg and foot.
4) Zuqiaoyin (GB 44)
Location: on the lateral side of the 4th toe, about 0.1 cun posterior to the corner of the toenail.
Indications: one-side headache, ophthalmalgia, pain in the hypochondriac region, febrile diseases, etc.
5) Zhiyin (UB 67)
Location: on the lateral side of the top of the digitus minimus about 0.1 cun proximal to the corner of the toenail.
Indications: headache, neck pain, retention labour, abnormal presentation.

37. What is the relation between Qi and blood?

Answer: Blood are Qi are closely related, the formation and circulation of blood depending upon Qi, whose formation and distribution are related to blood. Clinically, deficiency of Qi often leads to deficiency of blood, and deficiency of blood, in turn, often results in deficiency of Qi. Stagnation of Qi often causes stagnation of blood, and stagnation of blood, in turn, often causes stagnation of Qi.

38. Which channels distribute to the mouth?

Answer: Among the fourteen channels, the Du, Ren, liver, stomach and large intestine channels distribute to the mouth.

39. What points do the spots marked out in Fig. 11 stand for?

Answer: 1 stands for Ermen; 2 stands for Tinggong; 3 Stands for Tinghui.

40. Refer to proportional measurement, correct the mistakes occurring in the following figures (when necessary).

Answer: 1) The distance from the sternocostal angle to the centre of the umbili-

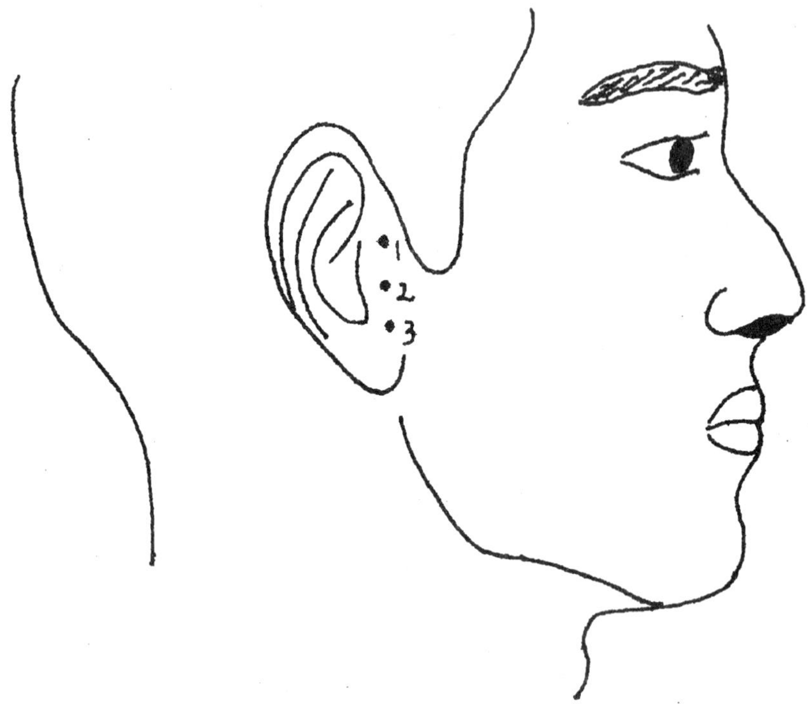

Fig. 11

cus is measured as 8 cun.

2) The distance from the prominence of the great trochanter to the middle of the patella is 19 cun.

3) The distance between the end of the axillary fold and the transverse cubital crease is 9 cun.

4) The distance between the transverse cubital crease and the transverse carpal crease is 12 cun.

5) The breadth of the four fingers close together at the level of the skin crease of the proximal interphalangeal joint at the dorsum of the middle finger is taken as 3 cun.

41. What are the main symptoms of Bi (obstacle) syndrome? What are the main criteria for the classification of wandering Bi, painful Bi, fixed Bi and febrile Bi? And what are the therapeutic principles and in particular what kind of manipulation should be performed for each of them?

Answer: The main symptom of Bi syndromes is arthralgia. There may be mus-

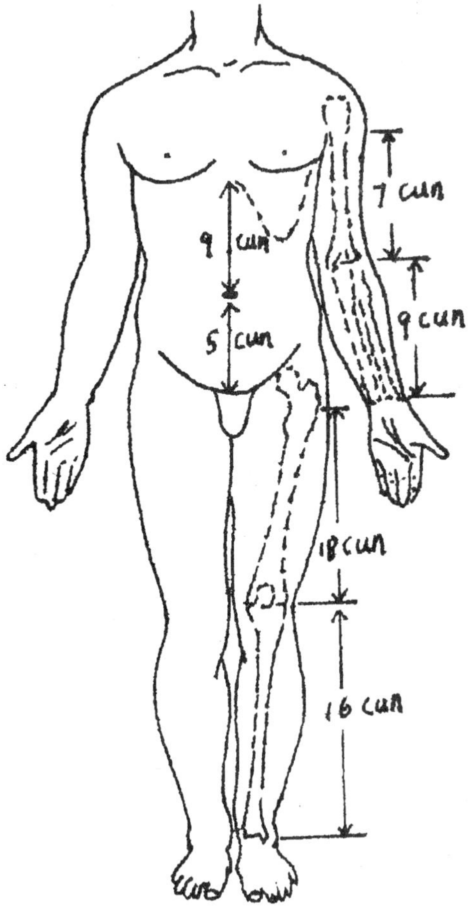

Fig. 12

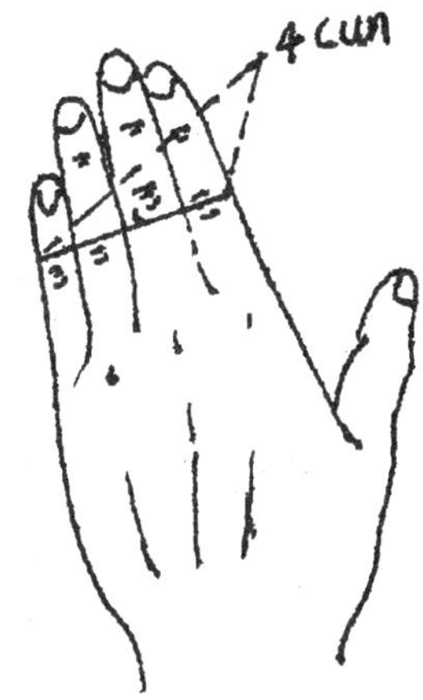

Fig. 13

cular soreness and numbness. In prolonged cases, contracture of the extremities, or even swelling or deformity of the joints may be present. Wandering Bi is characterized by wandering pain of the joint of the extremities with limitations of movement . Painful Bi usually responds to warmth and is aggravated by cold. There is no local inflammation.

Fixed Bi is characterized by arthralgia with fixed pain, attacks provoked by cloudy or wet weather.

Febrile Bi is characterized by arthralgia with local redness, swelling and tenderness in which one or several joints are involved.

Local and distal points are selected from the yang channels supplying the diseased areas for the purpose of eliminating wind, cold and damp. Wandering Bi is mainly treated with needling; painful Bi with moxibustion and needling as adjuvant. For severe pain, the use of intradermal needles or indirect moxibustion with ginger is recommended. Fixed Bi is treated with both acupuncture and moxibustion. Warming needle is also advisable. Febrile Bi is usually treated by needling with reducing method. Points are selected according to the courses of channels to relax the tension, remove obstacle from channels and collaterals, regulate Qi and blood and eliminate pathogenic factors.

42. What are the therapeutic properties of the five-Shu points?

Answer: Jing-Well points are indicated in mental illness and a stifling sensation in the chest, Ying-Spring points in febrile diseases, Shu-Stream points in Bi syndrome caused by pathogenic wind and damp, Jing-River point in asthma, cough, and sore throat, and He-Sea points in disorders of the intestines, stomach and the other Fu organs.

43. What do Ahshi points mean?

Answer: Ahshi points are tender spots or sensitive spots present in certain diseases. They have neither definite locations nor names. *Neijing* describes them:"Where there is a painful spot, there is an acupuncture point."

44. Take the treatment of syndromes of the heart as an example to show the application of the Yuan-Source and Luo-Conneciting points.

Answer: Clinically, Yuan and Luo points are used coordinately more than separately. When a channel is affected, the Yuan point of that channel may be chosen as the main point, while the Luo point of its externally-internally related channel combines with it to enhance the result. For instance, if the heart channel is affected, Shenmen (H 7), the Yuan point of the heart channel, and Zhizheng (SI 7), the Luo point of the small intestine channel, may be prescribed.

45. What does "reinforcing the 'mother' for deficiency syndrome and reducing the 'son' for excess syndrome" mean?

Answer: According to this principle, which points should be selected in dealing with deficiency and excess syndromes of the liver channel?

Answer: The mother point of a channel has a tonifying effect and is indicated in deficiency syndrome of its related channel; while the son point has a reducing effect and is indicated in the excess syndrome of its related channel. Hence the maxim: Reinforce the mother for deficiency syndrome and reduce the son for excess syndrome. In the light of this, when the liver channel is involved in deficiency syndrome, then the reinforcing method on Ququan (Liv 8) should be prescribed . On the other hand, in excess syndrome, Xingjian (Liv 2) with reducing method should be prescribed.

46. Describe briefly the pathway and main indications of the lung channel of Hand-Taiyin.

Answer: The lung channel of Hand-Taiyin orginates in the stomach, running downward to communicate with the large intestine. Turning back from the

intestine, it runs along the upper orifice of the stomach, then passes upward through the diaphragm to enter its pertaining organ, the lung. From the area between the lung and the throat, it comes out transversely to the region below the axilla. Then, it runs along the radial border of the anteiror aspect of the upper arm and passes in front of the heart channel of Hand-Shaoyin and the pericardium channel of Hand -Jueyin, then descends through the middle portion of the elbow to the medial border of the styloid process of the radius along the radial border of the forearm. From the posterior aspect of the wrist, it goes to the thenar along its border and extends to the end of the radial aspect of the pollex.
Indications: Diseases of the chest, throat, trachea, nose and lung.

47. Which viscera are related to the heart channel?

Answer: The heart channel pertains to the heart to communicate with the small intestine and connects directly with the lung and kidney.

48. Describe the etiology of nocturnal enuresis.

Answer: The causative factor is insufficiency of the Qi of the kidney and debility of the urinary bladder in controlling urination.

49. What are the contraindications of moxibustion?

Answer: Moxibustion is contraindicated in high fever either due to exogenous factors or deficiency of yin. Scarring moxibustion is not suitable for the face and head for cosmetic reasons. It should neither be applied to the lower abdomen or sacral region of pregnant women.

50. How is lower back pain caused by deficiency of kidney Qi, cold-damp and blood stasis to be differentiated?

Answer: Lower back pain caused by deficiency of kidney Qi:

One set is insidious, and pain is mild but protracted, with lassitude and weakness of the lumbar region and knee. Symptoms are intensifid after strain and stress and alleviated by bed rest.

Lower back pain caused by cold-damp:

Lower back pain usually occurs after exposure to pathogenic wind, cold and damp. Clinical manifestations are heavy sensation and pain in the dorsolumbar region and stiffness of muscles, limiting extension and flexion of the back. The pain may reflex downward to the buttocks and lower extremities, and the affected area usually feels cold. Pain becomes intensified in cloudy and rainy days and can not be alleviated by bed rest. Lower back pain caused by blood stasis:

The patient has a history of sprain of the lumbar region. Clinical manifestations are rigidity and pain of the lower back. The pain is fixed and aggravated on pressure and turning of the body.

51. What are the main manifestations of the syndrome of damp-heat in the urinary bladder?

Answer: The main manifestations are frequency and urgency of urination, difficult urination scanty in amount and with reddish tinge, and a burning pain in the urethra. There may be blood clots or stones in the urine, a red tongue with a yellow coating, and a fairly rapid pulse.

52. How are syndromes to be differentiated according to different taste in the mouth?

Answer: Tastelessness in the mouth usually indicates weakness of the spleen and stomach. Foul belching and acid regurgitation indicate retention of food. Stickiness and sweetish taste in the mouth show damp-heat in the spleen, while a bitter taste in the mouth points to hyperactivity of the fire of the liver and gallbladder.

53. What are the characteristics of the suprficial pulse, deep pulse, slow pulse and rapid pulse? What syndromes do they indicate respectively?

Answer: Superficial pulse responds to the finger when pressed lightly and becomes weak on heavy pressure. This pulse often occurs in the early stage of an exogenous disease, i.e. an exteiror syndrome. It may also occur in patients suffering from prolonged illness and who are in a state of general weakness.

Deep pulse means superficial palpation reveals no clear pulse, which is felt only upon heavy pressure. This often occurs in interior syndromes. Slow pulse refers to pulse with less than four beats per breath. This often occurs in cold syndromes. Rapid pulse refers to pulse with more than six beats per breath, a situation that often occurs in heat syndromes.

54. How is leukorrhea to be differentiated according to the colour of the discharge?

Answer: White discharge is usually due to deficiency of Qi and presence of damp. It is thin, whitish or yellowish, and with odour. Yellow discharge is due to downward infusion of damp-heat. It is pinkish or deep yellow and with fetid odour.

55. Describe the characteristics of syndromes caused by pathogenic wind.

Answer:

1) Wind, characterized by upward and outgoing dispersion, is a yang pathogenic factor. When it invades the body from outside, it often attacks the upper portion of the body, weakening the defensive Qi and causing derangement in the opening and closing of pores over the body surface. Clinical symptoms are headache,

nasal obstruction, soreness or itching of the throat, facial puffiness, aversion to wind, and sweating.

2) Wind occurs in gusts and is characterized by rapid change, pathogenic wind being espcially so.

3) Wind is characterized by constant movement.

4) Wind is apt to associate itself with other pathogenic factors.

56. In what organs are disorders caused by the seven emotional factors mainly seen?

Answer: The seven emotional factors usually affect the heart, liver and spleen. Excessive joy or fear and fright may cause mental restlessness and give rise to palpitation, insomnia, irritability, anxiety and even mental disorders. Excessive anger may cause dysfunction of the liver in promoting unrestraint and patency of vital energy and give rise to pain and distention in the costal and hypochondriac region, irregular menstruation, mental depression and irascibility Excessive grief, melancholy and meditation may cause dysfunction of the spleen and stomach in transportation and transformation and cause anorexia and abdominal fullness and distention after meals.

APPENDIXES

Standard Acupuncture Nomenclature

Part 1 Revised Edition

Points of Lung Meridian, LU.
Shoutaiyin Feijing xue

LU 1	Zhongfu	LU 7	Lieque
LU 2	Yunmen	LU 8	Jingqu
LU 3	Tianfu	LU 9	Taiyuan
LU 4	Xiabai	LU 10	Yuji
LU 5	Chize	LU 11	Shaoshang
LU 6	Kongzui		

Points of Large Intestine Meridian, LI.
Shouyangming Dachangjing xue

LI 1	Shangyang	LI 12	Zhouliao
LI 2	Erjian	LI 13	Shouwuli
LI 3	Sanjian	LI 14	Binao
LI 4	Hegu	LI 15	Jianyu
LI 5	Yangxi	LI 16	Jugu
LI 6	Pianli	LI 17	Tianding
LI 7	Wenliu	LI 18	Futu
LI 8	Xialian	LI 19	Kouheliao*
LI 9	Shanglian		Heliao#
LI 10	Shousanli	LI 20	Yingxiang
LI 11	Quchi		

*# Either of these can be used.

Points of Stomach Meridian, ST.
Zuyangming Weijing xue

ST 1	Chengqi	ST 24	Huaroumen
ST 2	Sibai	ST 25	Tianshu
ST 3	Juliao	ST 26	Wailing
ST 4	Dicang	ST 27	Daju
ST 5	Daying	ST 28	Shuidao
ST 6	Jiache	ST 29	Guilai
ST 7	Xiaguan	ST 30	Qichong
ST 8	Touwei	ST 31	Biguan
ST 9	Renying	ST 32	Futu
ST 10	Shuitu	ST 33	Yinshi
ST 11	Qishe	ST 34	Liangqiu
ST 12	Quepen	ST 35	Dubi
ST 13	Qihu	ST 36	Zusanli
ST 14	Kufang	ST 37	Shangjuxu
ST 15	Wuyi	ST 38	Tiaokou
ST 16	Yingchuang	ST 39	Xiajuxu
ST 17	Ruzhong	ST 40	Fenglong
ST 18	Rugen	ST 41	Jiexi
ST 19	Burong	ST 42	Chongyang
ST 20	Chengman	ST 43	Xiangu
ST 21	Liangmen	ST 44	Neiting
ST 22	Guanmen	ST 45	Lidui
ST 23	Taiyi		

Points of Spleen Meridian, SP.
Zutaiyin Pijing xue

SP 1	Yinbai	SP 12	Chongmen
SP 2	Dadu	SP 13	Fushe
SP 3	Taibai	SP 14	Fujie
SP 4	Gongsun	SP 15	Daheng
SP 5	Shangqiu	SP 16	Fu'ai
SP 6	Sanyinjiao	SP 17	Shidou
SP 7	Lougu	SP 18	Tianxi
SP 8	Diji	SP 19	Xiongxiang
SP 9	Yinlingquan	SP 20	Zhourong
SP 10	Xuehai	SP 21	Dabao
SP 11	Jimen		

Points of Heart Meridian, HT.
Shoushaoyin Xinjing xue

HT 1	Jiquan	HT 6	Yinxi
HT 2	Qingling	HT 7	Shenmen
HT 3	Shaohai	HT 8	Shaofu
HT 4	Lingdao	HT 9	Chaochong
HT 5	Tongli		

Points of Small Intestine Meridian, SI.
Shoutaiyang Xiaochangjing xue

SI 1	Shaoze	SI 11	Tianzong
SI 2	Qiangu	SI 12	Bingfeng
SI 3	Houxi	SI 13	Quyuan
SI 4	Wangu	SI 14	Jianwaishu
SI 5	Yanggu	SI 15	JIanzhongshu
SI 6	Yanglao	SI 16	Tianchuang
SI 7	Zhizheng	SI 17	Tianrong
SI 8	Xiaohai	SI 18	Quanliao
SI 9	Jianzhen	SI 19	Tinggong
SI 10	Naoshu		

Points of Bladder Meridian, BL.
Zutaiyang Pangguangjing xue

BL 1	Jingming	BL 35	Huiyang
BL 2	Cuanzhu (Zanzhu)	BL 36	Chengfu
BL 3	Meichong	BL 37	Yinmen
BL 4	Qucha (Quchai)	BL 38	Fuxi
BL 5	Wuchu	BL 39	Weiyang
BL 6	Chengguang	BL 40	Weizhong
BL 7	Tongtian	BL 41	Fufen
BL 8	Luoque	BL 42	Pohu
BL 9	Yuzhen	BL 43	Gaohuang
BL 10	Tianzhu	BL 44	Shentang
BL 11	Dazhu	BL 45	Yixi
BL 12	Fengmen	BL 46	Geguan
BL 13	Feishu	BL 47	Hunmen
BL 14	Jueyinshu	BL 48	Yanggang

BL 15	Xinshu	BL 49	Yishe
BL 16	Dushu	BL 50	Weicang
BL 17	Geshu	BL 51	Huangmen
BL 18	Ganshu	BL 52	Zhishi
BL 19	Danshu	BL 53	Baohuang
BL 20	Pishu	BL 54	Zhibian
BL 21	Weishu	BL 55	Heyang
BL 22	Sanjiaoshu	BL 56	Chengjin
BL 23	Shenshu	BL 57	Chengshan
BL 24	Qihaishu	BL 58	Feiyang
BL 25	Dachangshu	BL 59	Fuyang
BL 26	Guanyuanshu	BL 60	Kunlun
BL 27	Xiaochangshu	BL 61	Pucan (Pushen)
BL 28	Pangguangshu	BL 62	Shenmai
BL 29	Zhonglushu	BL 63	Jinmen
BL 30	Baihuanshu	BL 64	Jinggu
BL 31	Shangliao	BL 65	Shugu
BL 32	Ciliao	BL 66	Zutonggu
BL 33	Zhongliao	BL 67	Zhiyin
BL 34	Xialiao		

Points of Kidney Meridian, KI.
Zushaoyin Shenjing xue

KI 1	Yongquan	KI 15	Zhongzhu
KI 2	Rangu	KI 16	Huangshu
KI 3	Taixi	KI 17	Shangqu
KI 4	Dazhong	KI 18	Shiguan
KI 5	Shuiquan	KI 19	Yindu
KI 6	Zhaohai	KI 20	Futonggu
KI 7	Fuliu	KI 21	Youmen
KI 8	Jiaoxin	KI 22	Bulang
KI 9	Zhubin	KI 23	Shenfeng
KI 10	Yingu	KI 24	Lingxu
KI 11	Henggu	KI 25	Shencang
KI 12	Dahe	KI 26	Yuzhong
KI 13	Qixue	KI 27	Shufu
KI 14	Siman		

Points of Pericardium Meridian, PC.
Shoujueyin Xinbaojing xue

PC 1	Tianchi	PC 6	Neiguan
PC 2	Tianquan	PC 7	Daling
PC 3	Quze	PC 8	Laogong
PC 4	Ximen	PC 9	Zhongchong
PC 5	Jianshi		

Points of Triple Energizer Meridian, TE.
Shoushaoyang Sanjiaojing xue

TE 1	Guanchong	TE 13	Naohui
TE 2	Yemen	TE 14	Jianliao
TE 3	Zhongzhu	TE 15	Tianliao
TE 4	Yangchi	TE 16	Tianyou
TE 5	Waiguan	TE 17	Yifeng
TE 6	Zhigou	TE 18	Chimai (Qimai)
TE 7	Huizong	TE 19	Luxi
TE 8	Sanyangluo	TE 20	Jiaosun
TE 9	Sidu	TE 21	Ermen
TE 10	Tianjing	TE 22	Erheliao*
TE 11	Qinglengyuan		Heliao#
TE 12	Xiaoluo	TE 23	Sizhukong

Points of Gallbladder Meridian, GB.
Zushaoyang Danjing xue

GB 1	Tongziliao	GB 23	Zhejin
GB 2	Tinghui	GB 24	Riyue
GB 3	Shangguan	GB 25	Jingmen
GB 4	Hanyan	GB 26	Daimai
GB 5	Xuanlu	GB 27	Wushu
GB 6	Xuanli	GB 28	Weidao
GB 7	Qubin	GB 29	Juliao
GB 8	Shuaigu	GB 30	Huantiao
GB 9	Tianchong	GB 31	Fengshi
GB 10	Fubai	GB 32	Zhongdu
GB 11	Touqiaoyin	GB 33	Xiyangguan

*# Either of these can be used.

GB 12	Wangu	GB 34	Yanglingquan
GB 13	Benshen	GB 35	Yangjiao
GB 14	Yangbai	GB 36	Waiqiu
GB 15	Toulinqi	GB 37	Guangming
GB 16	Muchuang	GB 38	Yangfu
GB 17	Zhengying	GB 39	Xuanzhong
GB 18	Chengling	GB 40	Qiuxu
GB 19	Naokong	GB 41	Zulinqi
GB 20	Fengchi	GB 42	Diwuhui
GB 21	Jianjing	GB 43	Xiaxi
GB 22	Yuanye	GB 44	Zuqiaoyin

Points of Liver Meridian, LR.
Zujueyin Ganjing xue

LR 1	Dadun	LR 8	Ququan
LR 2	Xingjian	LR 9	Yinbao
LR 3	Taichong	LR 10	Zuwuli
LR 4	Zhongfeng	LR 11	Yinlian
LR 5	Ligou	LR 12	Jimai
LR 6	Zhongdu	LR 13	Zhangmen
LR 7	Xiguan	LR 14	Qimen

Points of Governor Vessel, GV.
Dumai xue

GV 1	Changqiang	GV 15	Yamen
GV 2	Yaoshu	GV 16	Fengfu
GV 3	Yaoyangguan	GV 17	Naohu
GV 4	Mingmen	GV 18	Qiangjian
GV 5	Xuanshu	GV 19	Houding
GV 6	Jizhong	GV 20	Baihui
GV 7	Zhongshu	GV 21	Qianding
GV 8	Jinsuo	GV 22	Xinhui
GV 9	Zhiyang	GV 23	Shangxing
GV 10	Lingtai	GV 24	Shenting
GV 11	Shendao	GV 25	Suliao
GV 12	Shenzhu	GV 26	Shuigou
GV 13	Taodao	GV 27	Duiduan
GV 14	Dazhui	GV 28	Yinjiao

Points of Conception Vessel, CV.
Renmai xue

CV 1	Huiyin	CV 13	Shangwan
CV 2	Qugu	CV 14	Juque
CV 3	Zhongji	CV 15	Jiuwei
CV 4	Guanyuan	CV 16	Zhongting
CV 5	Shimen	CV 17	Tanzhong (Shanzhong)
CV 6	Qihai	CV 18	Yutang
CV 7	Yinjiao	CV 19	Zigong
CV 8	Shenque	CV 20	Huagai
CV 9	Shuifen	CV 21	Xuanji
CV 10	Xiawan	CV 22	Tiantu
CV 11	Jianli	CV 23	Lianquan
CV 12	Zhongwan	CV 24	Chengjiang

LIST OF EQUIVALENT ALPHABETIC CODES OF MERIDIAN NAMES

Meridian	Standard code*		Other alphabetic codes used**
1. Lung Meridian	LU	I	F L Lu P
2. Large Intestine Meridian	LI	II	CO Co DCh DI Di GI IC IG Li
3. Stomach Meridian	ST	III	E Est M Ma S St V W
4. Spleen Meridian	SP	IV	B BP LP MP P RP RT Rt Sp
5. Heart Meridian	HT	V	C H HE He Ht X
6. Small Intestine Meridian	SI	VI	Du ID IG IT Si XCh
7. Bladder Meridian	BL	VII	B B1 PG UB V VU
8. Kidney Meridian	KI	VIII	K Ki N NI Ni R RN Rn Sh
9. Pericardium Meridian	PC	IX	CS CX ECS EH HC Hc KS MC MdH P Pe XB
10. Triple Energizer Meridian	TE	X	DE T TB TH TR TW SC SJ 3E 3H

* This is part of the alphameric code element of the standard acupuncture nomenclature adopted at Scientific Group to Adopt a Standard International Acupuncture Nomenclature, 1989.

** Some of the alphabetic codes shown here have already been discarded but may still have been used in older documents. They have therefore been included in this list.

11. Gallbladder Meridian	GB	XI	D G Go VB VF
12. Liver Meridian	LR	XII	F G H LE Le Liv LIV LV L
13. Governor Vessel	GV	XIII	DM DU Du GG Go Gv LG Lg T TM VG Vg
14. Conception Vessel	CV	XIV	Co Cv J JM KG Kg REN Ren RM VC Vc

Standard Acupuncture Nomenclature

Part 2 Revised Edition

Basic Technical Terms of Acupuncture
Eight Extra Meridians
Extra Points
Scalp Acupuncture
Acupuncture Needles
Unit of Measurement

Standard Nomenclature of Basic Technical Terms of Acupuncture

There have been differences in the English nomenclature of basic technical terms of acupuncture. For instance, Jing was sometimes translated as "meridian," but at other times as "channel." Another example is Zhenjiuxue, which was translated as "acupuncture point" or "acupoint." The following standard nomenclature was adopted at the meeting held in Hong Kong in 1985:

Meridian	Jing
Collateral	Luo
Meridian and Collateral	Jingluo
Main Meridian	Zhengjing
Extra Meridian	Qijing
Meridian Point	Jingxue
Extra Point	Qixue
Acupuncture Point	Zhenjiuxue

Standard Nomenclature of Eight Extra Meridians

At the meeting in Hong Kong in 1985, after a careful and detailed study and debate, the nomenclature for eight extra meridians was adopted with the exception of "Chongmai."

The phrase "Eight Extra Meridians," which includes the Conception and Governor Vessel Meridians plus six extra meridians, was officially recognized as the corporate title of this group.

It was unanimously decided to omit the term "meridian" after Conception Vessel and Governor Vessel in order to standardize the nomenclature of the eight extra meridians.

The members were requested to find a suitable English equivalent for "Chongmai" and to report to the Third Regional Working Group.

At the meeting in Seoul in 1987, "Chongmai" was again discussed. Various names were proposed such as Infusion Vessel, Sea Vessel, Gush Vessel, Flush Vessel, Charging Vessel and Ancestral Vessel. Most of the suggestions referred to the description in Neijing (Canon of Medicine), i.e. "sea of the blood and gas. " Members from China, however, noted that it was impossible for them to find a suitable English equivalent.

After a lengthy discussion, the terms Charging, Flush, Gush and Infusion were grouped as one with similar meanings and, considering the alphanumeric code, it was decided to use Flush Vessel and the abbreviation FV, with a footnote "Further investigation of a more suitable English nomenclature might be necessary."

At the meeting in Geneva in 1989, "Chongmai" was discussed again together with the participants from regions other than WHO Western Pacific Region. Thoroughfare Vessel and Thoroughway Vessel were proposed as possible English equivalents. After lively and careful discussion, it was finally decided to use Thoroughfare Vessel with the abbreviation TV.

Thus, the nomenclature of the eight extra meridians is as follows:

Standard Nomenclature of Eight Extra Meridians

GV	Dumai	Governor Vessel
CV	Renmai	Conception Vessel
TV	Chongmai	Thoroughfare Vessel
BV	Daimai	Belt Vessel
YinHV	Yinqiaomai	Yin Heel Vessel
YangHV	Yangqiaomai	Yang Heel Vessel
YinLV	Yinweimai	Yin Link Vessel
YangLV	Yangweimai	Yang Link Vessel

Standard Nomenclature of Extra Points

At the Tokyo meeting in 1984, 31 extra points were adopted, all of which are those recorded in the medical classics and are widely used. At the Hong Kong meeting in 1985, 5 extra points and 12 new points were adopted using the following criteria:

(1) The points should be in common use.

(2) They must be clinically effective.

(3) They must have a clear anatomical location.

(4) They must be at least 0.5 cun away from a classical acupuncture point.

(5) If an extra point has the same name as an existing point, a prefix must be added to it.

At the Seoul meeting in 1987, a suitable nomenclature for all the 48 acupuncture points was discussed. After careful consideration, it was unanimously agreed that all points outside the 361 classical acupuncture points should be called Extra Points. This should include all new points introduced after 1901, including 12 new points adopted in Hong Kong, namely, Qiuhou, Shangyingxiang, Yiming, Dingchuan, Yaoyi, Xiazhishi, Yaotongdian Wailaogong, Lanwei, Dannang, Neixiyan and Xinei. Thus, all told, the Working Group adopted 48 extra points.

The alphanumeric code of these 48 extra points was then discussed. The following principles were established and the alphanumeric code was adopted.

(1) head, neck and trunk regions, from the higher to the lower level;

(2) upper and lower extremities, from the proximal to the distal level and, if at the same level, from the medial to the lateral.

The following standard nomenclature was adopted for the 48 extra points.

This was also adopted at the Geneva Meeting in 1989.

Standard Nomenclature of Extra Points

Points of the Head and Neck, HN.
Toujing xue

Ex-HN 1	Sishencong	Ex-HN 9	Neiyingxiang
*Ex-HN 2	Dangyang	Ex-HN 10	Juquan
Ex-HN 3	Yintang	Ex-HN 11	Haiquan
Ex-HN 4	Yuyao	Ex-HN 12	Jinjin
Ex-HN 5	Taiyang	Ex-HN 13	Yuye
Ex-HN 6	Erjian	*Ex-HN 14	Yiming
*Ex-HN 7	Qiuhou	*Ex-HN 15	Jingbailao
*Ex-HN 8	Shangyingxiang		

Points of the Chest and Abdomen, CA.
Xiongfu xue

Ex-CA 1 Zigong

Points of the Back, B.
Beibu xue

*Ex-B 1	Dingchuan	*Ex-B 6	Yaoyi
Ex-B 2	Jiaji	Ex-B 7	Yaoyan
*Ex-B 3	Weiwanxiashu	Ex-B 8	Shiqizhui
Ex-B 4	Pigen	Ex-B 9	Yaoqi
*Ex-B5	Xiazhishi		

Points of the Upper Extremities, UE.
Shangzhi xue

Ex-UE 1	Zhoujian	*Ex-UE 7	Yaotongdian
Ex-UE 2	Erbai	*Ex-UE 8	Wailaogong
Ex-UE 3	Zhongquan	Ex-UE 9	Baxie
Ex-UE 4	Zhongkui	Ex-UE 10	Sifeng
Ex-UE 5	Dagukong	Ex-UE 11	Shixuan
Ex-UE 6	Xiaogukong		

Points of the Lower Extremities, LE.
Xiazhi xue

*Ex-LE 1	Kuangu	*Ex-LE 7	Lanwei
Ex-LE 2	Heding	Ex-LE 8	Neihuaijian
*Ex-LE 3	Xinei	Ex-LE 9	Waihuaijian
*Ex-LE 4	Neixiyan	Ex-LE 10	Bafeng
Ex-LE 5	Xiyan	Ex-LE 11	Duyin
Ex-LE 6	Dannang	Ex-LE 12	Qiduan

Standard Nomenclature of Scalp Acupuncture

Scalp acupuncture theraphy, whereby diseases are treated by needling on certain areas of the head, has been employed in China since 1970. It is now becoming one of the therapeutic methods frequently used in many countries.

Scalp acupuncture has been developed on the basis of the traditional medicine system of acupuncture. Its points are closely related to the meridians, classical acupuncture points and the theory of internal organs. Thus its nommenclature should reflect the theory and characteristics of meridians and acupuncture points.

This nomenclature is formulated on the principle of selecting points on the meridians decided by the locations in various regions of the head in combination with the classical method of through-needling (needling from one point to reach another point or more points).

Like the classical points, the nomenclature of scalp acupuncture consists of three essential elements, namely, alphanumeric code, Chinese phonetic alphabet (Pin yin) names and Chinese characters. The corresponding English equivalent is also given.

The alphabetic code name of scalp acupuncture is MS, this code name being derived from the terms "micro-system" and "scalp points."

This nomenclature was adopted at the meeting in Tokyo in 1984 after a lengthy discussion.

At the Geneva meeting, this nomenclature was also adopted with the inclusion of suitable diagrams.

* Selected at the meeting in Hong Kong in 1985, the other 31 being selected at the meeting in Tokyo in 1984.

Standard Nomenclature of Scalp Acupuncture

MS 1 Ezhongxian
Middle Line of Forehead
1 cun long from GV 24 Shenting straight down along the meridian.

MS 2 Epangxian I
Lateral Line 1 of Forehead
1 cun long from BL 3 Meichong straight down along the meridian.

MS 3 Epangxian II
Lateral Line 2 of Forehead
1 cun long from GB 15 Toulinqi straight down along the meridian.

MS 4 Epangxian III
Lateral Line 3 of Forehead
1 cun long from the point 0.75 cun medial to ST 8 Touwei. Straight down

MS 5 Dingzhongxian
Middle Line of Vertex
From GV 20 Baihui to GV 21 Qianding along the midline of head.

MS 6 Dingnie Qianxiexian
Anterior Oblique Line of Vertex-Temporal
From Qianshencong (one of acupuncture points of EX-HN 1 Sishencong, 1 cun anterior to GV 20 Baihui obliquely to GB 6 Xuanli.)

MS 7 Dingnie Houxiexian
Posteiror Oblique Line of Vertex-Temporal
From GV 20 Baihui obliquely to GB 7 Qubin.

MS 8 Dingpangxian I
Lateral Line 1 of Vertex
1.5 cun lateral to Middle Line of Vertex, 1.5 cun long from BL 7 Tongtian backward along the meridian.

MS 9 Dingpangxian II
Lateral Line 2 of Vertex
2.25 cun lateral to Middle Line of Vertex
1.5 cun long from GB 17 Zhengying backward along the meridian.

MS 10 Nieqianxian
Anterior Temporal Line
From GB 4 Hanyan to GB 6 Xuanli.

MS 11 Niehouxian
Posterior Temporal Line
From GB 8 Shuaigu to GB 7 Qubin.

MS 12 Zhenshang Zhengzhongxian
Upper-Middle Line of Occiput
From GV 18 Qiangjian to GV 17 Naohu.

MS 13 Zhenshang Pangxian
Upper-Lateral Line of Occiput
0.5 cun lateral and parallel to Upper-Middle Line of Occiput.

MS 14 Zhenxia Pangxian
Lower-Lateral Line of Occiput
2 cun long from BL 9 Yuzhen straight down.

Standard Nomenclature of Acupuncture Needles

At the meeting in Seoul in 1987, after a lively discussion, the standard nomenclature of filiform needles was adopted and the method of measurement was decided. The standard nomenclature of the "nine classical needles" and modern needles was also proposed as follows:

Standard Nomenclature of Filiform Needles

handle	Zhenbing
root	Zhengen
body	Zhenti
tip	Zhenjian

The diameter is measured at the root and the length of the needle is measured from the root to the tip.

The unit of measurement is the millimetre.

Proposed Standard Nomenclature of the "Nine Classical Needles"

(1) Shear needle	Chanzhen
(2) Round-point needle	Yuanzhen
(3) Spoon needle	Chizhen
(4) Lance needle	Fengzhen
(5) Stiletto needle	Pizhen
(6) Round-sharp needle	Yuanlizhen
(7) Filiform needle	Haozhen
(8) Long needle	Changzhen
(9) Big needle	Dazhen

Proposed Standard Nomenclature of Modern Needles

(1) Three-edged needle	Sanlengzhen
(2) Ringheaded thumbtack needle	Qinzhen
(3) Intradermal needle	Pineizhen
(4) Dermal needle	Pifuzhen

Standard Nomenclature of the Unit of Measurement

At the Seoul meeting in 1987, the Working Group discussed the unit for location of meridians and acupuncture points. It was reported that different units and systems were in use. Some countries used the term "inch" or other equivalent units in English. However, most of the countries used the cun/Cun, or tsun/Tsun.

After a long discussion, it was decided to use the cun (non-italicized) as the standardized nomenclature for the unit.

It was also noted that there were two different ways of defining the cun. Therefore, it was decided that the following standard nomenclature should be used in each measurement method:

B-cun   Gudu Fencun   bone proportional cun
F-cun   Shouzhi Tongshencun   finger cun

The Working Group also discussed standardization of the measurement of parts of the body using the cun.

Thirty-six parts of the body mentioned in Neijing (Canon of Medicine) were reviewed one by one. The following criteria were used:

(1) Commonly used
(2) Easy to measure
(3) Clearly defined anatomically
(4) Not controversial among the members

Some controversial parts were left for further investigation.

Standard measurements of six parts of the body were adopted as follows:

(1) from the upper border of the Manubrium to the end of the body of the Sternum =9B-cun
(2) from the end of the body of the Sternum to the Umbilicus=8B-cun
(3) from the Umbilicus to the upper border of the Symphysis pubis = 5B-cun
(4) from the Medial Malleolus to the ground = 3B-cun
(5) from the greater Trochanter to the knee joint = 19B-cun
(6) from the knee joint to the prominence of Lateral Malleolus = 16B-cun

图书在版编目(CIP)数据

中国针灸测试:英文/陈悬,崔永强著 .
—北京:外文出版社,1997 重印
ISBN 7-119-01587-7

Ⅰ.中… Ⅱ.①陈… ②崔… Ⅲ.针灸疗法-试题-英文 Ⅳ.R245

中国版本图书馆 CIP 数据核字(97)第 16272 号

外文出版社网址:
http://www.flp.com.cn
外文出版社电子信箱:
info@flp.com.cn
sales@flp.com.cn

中国针灸测试
陈　悬　崔永强　著

*

©外文出版社
外文出版社出版
(中国北京百万庄大街 24 号)
邮政编码 100037
北京外文印刷厂印刷
中国国际图书贸易总公司发行
(中国北京车公庄西路 35 号)
北京邮政信箱第 399 号　邮政编码 100044
1993 年(16 开)第 1 版
1997 年第 1 版第 2 次印刷
2001 年第 1 版第 3 次印刷
(英)
ISBN 7-119-01587-7/R·95(外)
08000
14-E-2811S